The Singing Teacher's
Guide to

Transgender Voices

The Singing Teacher's Guide to

Transgender Voices

Liz Jackson Hearns, MM
Brian Kremer, MM

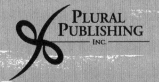

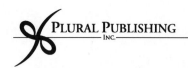

5521 Ruffin Road
San Diego, CA 92123

e-mail: info@pluralpublishing.com
website: http://www.pluralpublishing.com

Typeset in 11/13 Garamond by Flanagan's Publishing Services, Inc.
Printed in the United States of America by McNaughton & Gunn
20 19 18   2 3 4 5

Library of Congress Cataloging-in-Publication Data

Names: Jackson Hearns, Liz, author. | Kremer, Brian, author.
Title: The singing teacher's guide to transgender voices / Liz Jackson
  Hearns, MM, Brian Kremer, MM.
Description: San Diego, CA : Plural, [2018] | Includes bibliographical
  references and index.
Identifiers: LCCN 2018000653| ISBN 9781635500936 (alk. paper) | ISBN
  1635500931 (alk. paper)
Subjects: LCSH: Voice disorders--Treatment. | Communicative
  disorders—Treatment. | Voice culture—Complications.
Classification: LCC RF511.T73 H43 2018 | DDC 616.85/5606—dc23
LC record available at https://lccn.loc.gov/2018000653

In an attempt to maintain cohesiveness and simplicity, this text will use "transgender" as an umbrella term that encompasses any individual whose gender identity and/or gender expression differs from the sex and/or gender they were assigned at birth.

CONTENTS

PART THREE: The Experience

FOREWORD BY DAS JANSSEN, PhD

"Don't be silly."

"You'll grow out of it."

"What will people think?"

"Stop making mountains out of molehills."

"You'd be prettier if. . . ."

Or no words at all. Just that grim, embarrassed look some parents get when they introduce their kid to a coworker. The thin-lipped rigidity of a face refusing to see tears in the eyes of a child forced to look at the mirror over and over again during back-to-school-clothes shopping ordeals.

They don't always mean to gaslight us; it's really true that they don't understand just how it is their precious little daughter can be so adamant about being a boy. Or their handsome little man can long for a pretty dress. Or how their otherwise bright child can be so confused by demands to act like just one gender all the time. They changed our diapers after all; they know what they think is the truth. Sometimes their responses come from revulsion, but just as often, it's love; they're afraid for us. The world is not kind to people who are different and they want us safe.

So they shut us up. They teach us to hide and be quiet about the truth we know. They teach us to not make trouble, to control what we look at and say.

All. The. Time.

And then they decide that the eating disorders, the self-injury, the confused emotional outbursts are proof that we're intrinsically unstable, so they're less likely than ever to listen when we tell them the truth that contradicts what they think they know. We're not unstable; we're stressed.

Human beings are social animals. We need one another and we need to be heard. And we need to be heard as who and what we are. Another thing human beings need to do is sing, especially in community. This is why people still love to go to concerts in this age of recordings; it's why nearly every religion has some kind of communal singing: When we sing together, we create community. A certain manner of trust is forged when we sing together, and it is shattered when we are silenced. I still cringe at what I learned at age 7 when, as a newcomer to the church children's choir, I was told to mouth the words because I was too loud. Make no mistake, this was a gender thing: None of the other boys were expected to be ladylike and quiet.

We don't have to like everyone we sing with, but we do create communal experience by singing with them. One way a robust community is different from a group of friends is that communities include people we aren't friends with. We don't have the intimacy with every member of a community that we have to our circles of friends, but we're not strangers either. We pursue common goals at varying emotional distances, varying levels of like and dislike. Community functions as one middle gear between alienation and friendship, one of the many found in human relationships.

Those middle gears often get lost to people who have to hide who we are. There are people we trust (a tiny few) and people we don't trust (most people) and that's all there is. Other options are a luxury we don't have when we have to hide ourselves away. Communities of singers, people who literally raise their voices, can be fraught spaces. Traditional choirs gender-categorize singers even beyond notions of masculine and feminine (bass, alto, tenor, etc.), hammering the messages home: "You don't belong here," "We can't accommodate you," "The entire science of physics contradicts what you say about yourself." (Spoiler: not true)

This is why what Liz and Brian are doing with this book is so important. In studying trans voice health, including vocal physiology, tone, volume, pitch, breath, effects of hormone therapy, and all the other elements of voices and how we use them, they address a crucial need: Trans people need voices that make sense in the context we occupy today. We need to be heard. Whether we're singing or modifying speech habits to bring our voices into conformity with what makes sense in our particular lives, in this particular time, and in these particular cultures we inhabit, many of us have a voice for the first time when we receive trans-friendly and knowledgeable vocal training.

In my case, being lucky enough to have a trans-affirming voice teacher has helped me reestablish my natural state as a loudmouth who sings for the sheer pleasure of singing. After starting to take testosterone, I had to reassure a lot of people that I wasn't sick, just hoarse. I was going through puberty at age 44. It was clearly time for vocal training, and I asked about that at my neighborhood music store. Finding a trans-friendly voice teacher is a pretty rare thing. Luckily, they had just the person for me. My teacher was never intrusive with questions but always ready to chat and did the one thing so many people forget to do: listened to me. Really listened.

It's safe to say that most of us are not going to become overnight sensations, taking the world by storm and making vast fortunes as singers. Most of us are never going to pursue professional singing at all. And those who will? Well, they'll certainly be aided by the work Liz and Brian are doing: The more we understand about trans voice, the more voices of trans people we'll hear on the radio. For us ordinary trans mortals not destined for superstardom, the benefits of voice training are life-altering.

Voice training allows us to take some control of something we've been told we're helpless over our entire lives. The discipline of regular practice, yielding the results *we* need and desire, asserts our own agency. That is reinforced when we are taken seriously by the professionals who teach us. Our lessons and choir practices confirm that we are not hopelessly unintelligible and allow us to enter a broader range of community relationship with others.

Vocal training allows us to be heard as we really are in that wider community. Each of us has an imperfect body to work with, just like everyone else. Being able to set our own goals about how we want to be heard and learn how to achieve that also helps with coming to terms with the parts of ourselves that are more resistant to change. A healthy response is to find what we do like and can manage and work with those so we can continue to love ourselves. Dysphoria is a real thing, and singing is not therapy. But singing is one way of gaining the tools to find our own limitations, and happy surprises can help to undo some of the damage dysphoria does. We can say, "My lungs will probably never give me the boom I wish I could have, but hey, listen to how sweet it is in this range over here."

Trans-friendly and trans-competent music education engages us in a wider range of relationships with our own bodies and abilities as well as with other people. So listen to Liz and Brian. They're starting an important conversation, and there is a lot to be discussed and learned, not only about trans people and our voices but about human people's voices and our assumptions about who gets to be heard.

INTRODUCTION

It is in our nature as humans to categorize the sensory stimulants we receive into groups we are familiar with. Our ancestors needed to simplify their complex environments to ensure survival, and so separated objects into categories like blue or not-blue, water or not-water, one or the other. We make the same categorizations today about the people we encounter in our social environments. This person is old or young, tall or short, male or female. These categorizations happen immediately and subconsciously and are necessary for us as a species to help process the overwhelming amount of information we receive about our surroundings and encounters. The binary system is not always useful, however; there are innumerable of shades of blue, and each is meaningful in describing different objects. The same holds true for gender. Male and female are neither mutually exclusive, nor are they the only options available to describe a person. Gender, just like color, exists and is experienced along a spectrum.

In educating yourself to work with transgender singers, it is imperative to train your mind for flexibility. "Male" and "female" are intentionally put into quotations here to denote that these words may no longer have the concrete meaning that you traditionally assigned to them. As you explore the spectrum of gender identity, expression, and perception, you will begin to understand gender as a construct, a fallacy used to categorize whole humans into separable parts. You will notice the pervasiveness of the gender binary in our daily lives, from bathrooms and flight reservations to medical forms and clothing, even gender pronouns of deities. If you are ready to serve and guide your students in transgender and gender nonconforming communities, you may need to let go of previous ways of thinking about gender and see the world in a totally new way.

Before we attempt to digest the lives and experiences of transgender people, let's get clear about that word, *transgender*. It is an adjective to describe someone whose assigned and experienced gender are not the same—not necessarily opposite, but not the same. When you talk about transgender people, language is paramount because you are describing a group of multifaceted individuals in terms of one tiny aspect of themselves. As with any marginalized group of people, we see them for the nameable things they struggle with, but we must see them as whole, as well. These are individuals with rich lives and a variety of experiences and interests that have nothing to do with gender, so when we talk about transgender people in no other terms than their gender identity and expression, we owe it to them to at least be accurate and respectful about it.

The decision to support and teach transgender singers is not as simple as just taking on another student. We must start by noticing our own gender biases and begin to separate the sounds a voice can make with the gender identity of the singer. Our students need us to research into trans identity, trans issues, and the trans/gnc experience, so that we can meet them where they are, rather than ask them to be expert gender theorists for us. We need to offer evidence-based information about the physiological changes that sometimes accompany medical transition (if a singer decides to go through medical transition), which can affect vocal function in ways that might be different from what we are used to. We need to learn about the aspects of social and legal transition that affect our students, as well. We must put effort into creating a gender-inclusive learning environment where singers feel affirmed, welcomed, and respected.

The goal of the following text is to aid in the development of a successful vocal pedagogy for the training of transgender singers, help the academic community understand the needs of transgender students as it pertains to vocal training, and engage in a broader discussion about the presence of transgender students in lessons and classes and how this can improve teaching, curriculum, and classroom environments. It is hard to fathom the difficulty and daily stress trans people go through. We in the voice teaching community have so much catching up to do to serve and to understand our trans and nonbinary students and our fellow teachers who are trans and nonbinary. We have a responsibility to learn from trans voice teachers when we can and amplify the voices of our students when they are ready to be heard.

As you embark on your journey into guiding trans singers toward healthy, joyful singing, you will find yourself faced with new challenges, new sounds, and new ideas about gender and voice. Open yourself to those challenges, and create a singing studio where people with different gender identities and expressions have a welcoming, open space in which to express themselves through singing. Know that by revealing themselves to you, they are fighting against a lifetime of disappearing. See your students, hear them, learn about them, but remember that the person standing in front of you is complete already and that their gender identity and expression are only parts of that whole person. They have come to you to unveil, discover, and claim their true voice and you have a precious opportunity to help them find confidence and strength in that process. Practice patience and compassion, and the willingness to be equally visible yourself. To earn the trust of a transgender person enough for them to turn over their voice is a powerfully humbling experience, and hopefully this text will start you on the path in this rewarding, life-changing work.

ACKNOWLEDGMENTS

Liz:

Thank you, Sean, for your support and patience, and for making me feel like a superhero while this book took over our weekends and living room tables. Das, thank you for constantly challenging me, from that first coffee shop conversation where you asked me, "What is gender?" to holding me and walking with me through my own journey. Thank you, Kelly, for your mentorship and solidarity, and for giving openly your experience and expertise. Thank you to friends and family, and to my colleagues at The Voice Lab for cheering me on and helping us continue to grow in service to trans and nonbinary singers. Thank you, Brian, for your partnership and friendship; your deep passion and enthusiasm are inspiring and infectious, and I am so excited for what lies ahead with this project. And to my students, especially the four of you who shared so generously in your interviews, I am immeasurably grateful. You surprise and delight me, and because of you, I see and hear the world in new ways every day. I have learned so much from you, and I am deeply honored to be a fellow traveler with you.

Brian:

I would like to thank my wife Jen and daughter Harley for their constant love and support and for allowing me the time to write this book. To my mother, Melinda, whose beautiful coloratura soprano voice inspired me as a child as it rang through the house and whose kind and generous spirit lifts those around her. To my father Stuart and sister Jenna, I hope that you are together somewhere, singing, dancing, driving cars, riding motorcycles, and swimming with the dolphins. I am grateful for the time we had together and love you both very much. To all the family, friends, students, and colleagues who have been with me along this process, thank you for your encouragement, curiosity, ideas, and motivation. Thank you, Elon University and University of the Arts, for supporting this research. Lastly, thank you, Liz, for being an amazing and brilliant research partner and friend.

We would like to give a special thanks to Katja Tetzlaff and Gene Knific for their contributions with illustrations and graphics.

PART ONE

The Person

CHAPTER

1

Deconstructing Gender

Gender is like a Rubik's Cube with one hundred squares per side, and every time you twist it to take a look at another angle, you make it that much harder a puzzle to solve.

—Sam Killermann, *A Guide to Gender: The Social Justice Advocate's Hanbook* (p. 169)

INTRODUCTION

Nowhere else in the musical arts are gender roles as staunchly established and upheld as in voice. The binary gender system presides over voice parts, repertoire choices, role casting, competitions, costuming, dressing rooms, and more. Because the established social gender roles of singers have never been deconstructed or recalibrated, the prevalence of the binary system is so ingrained that it often goes unnoticed until someone who does not fit into the system disrupts it. That disruption leaves many voice teachers and music educators at a loss for means to guide their students in ways that support them artistically and help build their careers in such a heavily gendered environment. Voice teachers strive to acquire and demonstrate the skills and knowledge to help any student who wants it, but pedagogy for gender diverse singers—those whose identity and experience lie outside the established norms—is likely not part of the teacher's training. Many voice teachers have little or no experience working with transgender or gender nonconforming singers and so may feel reluctant at the prospect. This lack of competency and resultant lack of motivation to build competency in teaching transgender students creates a major obstacle for these singers who are in pursuit of voice training.

Deconstructing gender requires teachers and students alike to reevaluate gender roles in order to create a space where all gender identities, and expression of those identities through singing, are valid and important. In this way, teachers begin to develop trans-competency and work to reduce the myriad cultural and linguistic barriers between voice teachers and the transgender community that interfere with effective and accessible voice training. Trans-competency impacts the entire voice studio for all students, across the entire gender spectrum, and allows educators to dismantle and rebuild relationships between gender and voice in healthy and empowering ways.

The vocabulary, tools, and scenarios in this chapter may challenge years of profoundly deep-rooted beliefs but will broaden gender comprehension and hopefully compassion alongside it. This chapter demonstrates the differences between a person's sex and gender, delineates the factors that form one's gender identity, outlines both affirming and problematic LGBTQ+ terminology, and explores the unique and complex vulnerability that transgender students face in voice training.

GENDER VERSUS SEX

It has long been tradition to use the terms *sex* and *gender* interchangeably, but these two terms are not inherently linked. Understanding the difference between *sex* and *gender* is a significant step toward trans-competency and to working with transgender and gender nonconforming or nonbinary singers. *Sex* describes the biological differences between people, both anatomical and physiological. *Gender*, on the other hand, is behavioral, not biological. It is experienced and perceived, not absolute (Jones, 2009). It is uniquely individual to each person.

Sex is assigned at birth based on genetic chromosomes, hormone levels, primary sex characteristics, and secondary sex characteristics. There are two sex chromosomes in humans: X and Y. These sex chromosomes form one of the 23 pairs of human chromosomes in each cell of the body (Gilbert, 2009). Typically, babies assigned female at birth have two X chromosomes and babies assigned male at birth have one X and one Y chromosome. This can vary, as there are cases of both male- and female-assigned babies with other combinations of the X and Y chromosomes (Botswick & Martin, 2007; Jones, 2009). Hormones also influence an individual's assigned sex. In most cases, female-assigned infants have higher amounts of estrogen and progesterone than testosterone, while male-assigned infants have higher amounts of testosterone than estrogen or progesterone (Jones, 2009). Primary and secondary sex characteristics include reproductive organs that are present at birth and characteristics that develop during adolescence, including facial and body hair, changes in body shape, and changes in voice (Gilbert, 2000).

Whereas sex is assigned at birth, *gender* is self-determined by the individual. Through behavioral observation, societies begin to establish gender as a set of standards that determines the attitudes, gestures, and other characteristics typically associated with being mostly male or mostly female (Dragowski, Scharrón-del Río, & Sandigorsky, 2011). Children learn to perform aspects of their assigned gender from their communities and to fulfill expectations from their peers, parents, neighbors, families, and social groups (The Trevor Project, 2013). For some, those aspects are congruent with the gender they know themselves to be. For others, gender roles and expectations around hairstyle, wardrobe, makeup, vocabulary, gestures, interests and passions, or general attitudes are incongruent with their self-experienced gender or how they wish to express their gender within their own societal structures. The term *transgender* describes someone who experiences this incongruence between assigned sex and self-experienced gender identity.

Once establishing *sex* as biological and *gender* as behavioral, each individual gains the freedom to determine their own gender identity regardless of their assigned birth sex. This is in contrast to a flawed yet deeply ingrained binary gender system wherein each person is recognized as only one of two genders: male or female. This binary system does not allow for variance between one's assigned sex and their experienced gender identity and greatly limits gender to a set of characteristics determined by outdated standards rather than a genuine, idiosyncratic expression of authentic identity.

Gender Identity, Expression, and Perception

In order to define gender, we must explore the complicated relationship between gender identity, gender expression, and gender perception. It may seem easy to take for granted, but each person exhibits these three points within the tapestry of gender. Simply, gender identity is "who I am," gender expression is "how I show it," and gender perception is "how I am seen."

Gender identity is one's own internal, personal sense of being a man, woman, both, neither, or other nonbinary identity. Choosing language to describe personal gender identity might include transgender, bigender, gender fluid, gender nonconforming, gender questioning, genderqueer, nonbinary, two-spirit, cisgender, or another term.

Gender expression is the external presentation of someone's gender identity, usually through masculine, feminine, or gender variant behavior. These are factors such as clothing, mannerisms, hairstyle, vocal quality, and body characteristics. Gender expression can be congruent with one's gender identity, but it is sometimes separate from, or not related to, one's gender identity. An individual might choose to express themselves in a way that is in contrast to what society would assume is typical for that gender. For folks in *transition*, or in the process of aligning their gender expression with their gender identity, they may choose gender-variant means of expression for safety reasons or to ease the stress and burden of social and/or medical transition.

Gender perception is how society and the world perceives, observes, or reacts to another's gender expression and/or identity. It is normal to categorize information about someone's gender based on the way they express themselves. Gender perception influences how easily a gender diverse person moves through the world from ordering coffee to taking the stage. Assuming another person's gender identity from initial outward perception, based on interpretation of their gender expression, is tenuous and potentially offensive. It is imperative to allow individuals to reveal their gender identity, or simply ask for their preferred pronouns, rather than assuming. This is good advice not just as a voice teacher but also as a fellow gender-conscious human being.

Gender perception plays a direct role in the voice studio as well as in daily life. The voice, being a secondary sex characteristic, is often used to categorize people. For example, even in a brief telephone conversation, the listener immediately begins making assumptions about their conversation partner. This includes age, ethnicity, where the speaker lives or was raised (accent), level of intelligence, and gender. The sound of a voice is deeply tied to its perception by others.

For some transgender individuals, the external sound of their voice doesn't align with how they wish to express their gender identity. An uneasiness or detachment from the sound of one's own voice, called *vocal dysphoria*, can be common. This can lead to overwhelming anxiety about using voice in everyday speaking, especially in singing.

Some students pursue voice training as a way to change the way they're perceived by others and some do not. When teaching transgender and gender nonconforming singers, it is important not to assume their desired vocal timbre, quality, or range based on immediate perception of their gender identity. Discuss with the student to learn about their desired vocal range and quality, and offer expertise and counsel as to whether it is possible based on the physical characteristics and limitations of the vocal mechanism.

How we perceive another person's gender emerges subconsciously from the way they choose to express themselves. The way they choose to express themselves is sometimes, though not always, connected to their gender identity. Once we realize that we are all diverse in our behaviors, emotions, interests, and mannerisms and that we all interpret differently the same traits in others, we begin to grasp how logical it is that there must be more than two gender choices. This space, the out-of-bounds of this two-gender system, can be called *the gender spectrum.*

The Gender Spectrum

The most difficult decision when painting a room is selecting the color. Amid the various color swatches available at the hardware store, delineating color without expert eyes can be a daunting challenge. The desired color range might be blue, but is it raindrop blue, Missoula blue, wave crest blue, antique blue, cobalt, periwinkle, aqua? Where is the line, exactly, between blue and the other colors? What seems simple is actually diverse and nuanced; each shade of blue is beautiful and distinctive in its own way. Attempting to describe each distinct hue as *blue* or *not blue* is inadequate, just as it is inadequate to describe a person's identity as either male or female. These two identities are neither mutually exclusive, nor are they the only options available to describe a person. Gender, just like color, exists and is experienced along a spectrum.

Sam Killermann, social justice comedian and author of *A Guide to Gender* (2017b), explains the gender spectrum through a system he calls The Genderbread Person, shown in Figure 1–1. The Genderbread Person illustrates the ways in which gender identity, gender expression, sexual orientation, and birth-assigned sex vary in each person, living continuously on a sliding scale (Killermann, 2017a). It shows identity as being rooted in one's brain, expression executed outwardly, and sex associated with some parts of the body. It is also worth noting that there is a separation of romantic and sexual attraction from gender. Gender identity is not equal to or inextricably linked to sexual orientation or romantic attraction.

According to a recent study using diffusion-weighted magnetic resonance imaging, gender diversity can be observed through brain structure and chemistry. Upon comparing white matter in the brains of cisgender females, cisgender males, transgender females, and transgender males, Kranz (2014) concludes, "white matter microstructure in [transgender males] and [transgender females] falls halfway between that of [cisgender females] and [cisgender males]" (Kranz et al., 2014, p. 15474) This is the magnificence of the gender spectrum. Instead of an inadequate and inaccurate binary system based on gender stereotypes and biased assumptions, there is evidence of

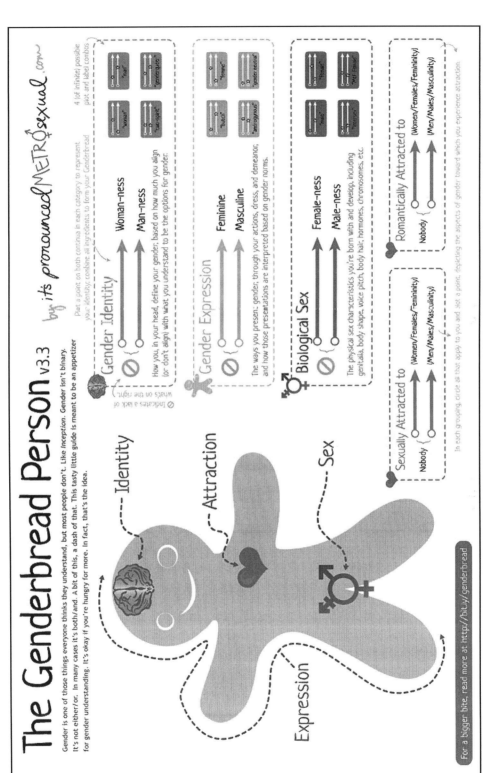

Figure 1-1. The Genderbread Person. Public Domain.

a beautiful, complex, and diverse spectrum of human identities, behaviors, and interests that represents a truer and more nuanced model of human gender.

TERMS AND VOCABULARY FOR LGBTQIA+ IDENTITIES

The following is a compilation of LGBTQ+ terminology to include and define the most essential terms, abbreviations, colloquialisms, and phrases available at this point in time that teachers should know when working toward cultural competency. It is important to note, however, that these terms merely reflect current cultural and societal norms in Western and American societies. Other factors likely influence the identity of a LGBTQ+ individual, including race/ethnicity, religion, ability, language, or socioeconomic status. Because of these factors, it should not be assumed that the definitions below are generalizable to all LGBTQ+ identities.

Advocate: 1. /*noun*/ a person who actively works to educate themselves and others about marginalized groups and uses that education to diminish intolerance and mistreatment and support social equality. 2. /*verb*/ to speak, plea, argue in favor of, or support a cause; the act of working to end intolerance, dehumanization, and mistreatment of marginalized groups.

Agender: /*adj.*/ describes a person for whom there is very little or no connection to the traditional systems of gender, or whose gender identity is neither male nor female, that they are without gender.

Ally: /*noun*/ a person, typically cisgender and/or heterosexual, who supports and advocates for the lesbian, gay, bisexual, transgender, queer + communities.

Androgyny/Androgynous /*adj.*/ 1. exhibiting both male and female characteristics. 2. an expression of gender through clothing, hairstyle, or appearance that has both feminine and masculine elements. Not typically a term of self-identity.

Androsexual/Androphilic: /*adj.*/ describes a person who is romantically, sexually, and/or emotionally attracted to men and/or masculinity.

AFAB /*adj.*/ acronym for "assigned female at birth."

AMAB /*adj.*/ acronym for "assigned male at birth."

Aromantic: /*adj.*/ describes a person for whom there is "little or no romantic attraction to others and/or has a lack of interest in romantic relationships/behavior. Sometimes abbreviated to 'aro' (pronounced like 'arrow')" (Killermann, 2017b, p. 258).

Asexual: /*adj.*/ describes a person who experiences little or no sexual attraction or lack of sexual interest in others. Sometimes abbreviated to "ace."

Bicurious: /*adj.*/ describes a person who is curious about their attraction to people of the same gender or may be questioning their sexual and/or romantic orientation.

Bigender: /*adj.*/ describes a person whose gender identity fluctuates between male or mostly male and female or mostly female, identifying with both genders and sometimes a third gender.

Biological sex: /*noun*/ a medical term that describes anatomical, chromosomal, and hormonal characteristics. This term can be problematic because of its historical use to describe someone's assigned gender when in fact, biological iterations of sex and/or gender are diverse and unique for each person.

Biphobia: /*noun*/ 1. harmful or negative attitudes expressed toward bisexual individuals, including fear, anger, erasure, or resentment. 2. **Biphobic:** /*adj.*/ describes an individual who harbors negative attitudes toward bisexual individuals.

Birth-Assigned Sex: /*noun*/ "the classification of people as male, female or intersex. At birth, infants are assigned a sex based on a combination of bodily characteristics including: chromosomes, hormones, internal reproductive organs, genitals, and an expectation to develop specific secondary sex characteristics. In our society, sex is normatively categorized into male and female, although variation in sex is natural and frequent" (The Trevor Project, 2013).

Bisexual: /*adj.*/ describes people who are physically, emotionally, and/or romantically attracted to both men and women, or more than one gender.

Butch: / *noun* & *adj.* / "a person who identifies themselves as masculine, whether it be physically, mentally or emotionally. 'Butch' is sometimes used as a derogatory term for lesbians, but has also been claimed as an affirmative identity label" (Killermann, 2017b, p. 260).

Chest Binder: /*noun*/ a compression tank undergarment that minimizes the appearance of breasts and contours the torso to appear less feminine; used when chest binding.

Chest Binding: /*verb*/ the act of minimizing the appearance of breasts by using a compression tank called a chest binder.

Chest Reconstruction Surgery: /*noun*/ 1. double mastectomy to create a more masculine and/or less feminine chest. (see "Top Surgery") 2. Breast implants or other surgical option for feminization of the contour of the chest.

Cisgender /*adj.*/ describes a person for whom the personal experience of their gender is congruent with the gender they were assigned at birth. Often abbreviated as "cis."

Cisnormativity: /*noun*/ the assumption that all people are cisgender, which leads to erasure and invisibility of transgender and gender-diverse (noncisgender) identities.

Cissexism: /*noun*/ behaviors that grant preferential treatment to cisgender people, rising from the assumption or belief that cisgender identities are more natural or correct than gender-diverse identities.

Closeted: /*adj.*/ describes an individual who is not open or public about their queer sexuality or identity, either by their own choice or out of necessity for their safety or fear of rejection from family, employers, and so on. Also known as being "in the closet."

Coming Out: /*verb*/ 1. personally, the process of accepting one's own sexuality and/or gender identity. 2. for friends, family, and community, the process of sharing or disclosing one's sexuality and/or gender identity with others.

Cross-Dressing: /*verb*/ to wear clothes of another gender/sex; a form of gender expression.

Drag: /*noun*/ the act of dressing in gendered clothing and adopting gendered behavior and mannerisms as part of a performance whether for entertainment or political commentary.

Dyke: /*noun*/ "referring to a masculine presenting lesbian. While often used derogatorily, it can be adopted affirmatively by many lesbians (both more masculine and more feminine presenting lesbians) as a positive self-identity term" (Killermann, 2017b, p. 261).

Electrolysis: /*noun*/ a beauty regimen to reduce the appearance of facial hair.

Facial Feminization Surgery: /*noun*/ a series or combination of plastic surgeries to reshape the forehead, nose, jaw, chin, lips, cheeks, ears, or other parts of the face to appear more feminine. Often abbreviated to "FFS."

Fag(got): /*noun*/ "derogatory term referring to a gay person, or someone perceived as queer. Occasionally used as a self-identifying affirming term by some gay men, at times in the shortened form 'fag'" (Killermann, 2017b, p. 262).

Feminine-of-center: /*adj.*/ describes a person whose identity, presentation, or relationships to others reside in the range of feminine but who does not necessarily identify as a woman.

Feminize: /*noun*/ the process of altering an aspect of presentation to be more feminine. This may include, but is not limited to, clothing, makeup, voice, or hormone therapy.

Femme: / *adj.* & *noun* / 1. describes a person who identifies as physically or mentally feminine. 2. a feminine-presenting queer person.

Fluid(ity): / *adj.*/ "generally with another term attached, like gender-fluid or fluid-sexuality, fluid(ity) describes an identity that may change or shift over time between or within the mix of the options available (e.g., man and woman, bi and straight)" (Killermann, 2017b, p. 262).

FtM: / *abbreviation* / stands for "female to male." Mostly used in a medical context and should be avoided because of the implication that a person goes *from* one gender *to* another, rather than having always identified as their affirmed gender.

Gay: /*adj.*/ 1. describes a person who is emotionally, physically, and/or sexually attracted to members of the same sex and/or gender.

Gender: /*noun*/ a set of behaviors, characteristics, gestures, emotional traits, attitudes, and social expectations that are associated with being mostly male or mostly female. Gender is constructed by the societies and communities that perpetuate it and varies between cultures and across time periods.

Gender Assignment: /*noun*/ similar to, but separate from, sex assignment. Once sex is assigned at birth, gender assignment and corresponding gender role expectations are enforced from birth regarding presentation, behavior, and activities or interests in which one may participate.

Gender Attribution: /*noun*/ the process by which someone assumes the gender of another person through their gender expression.

Gender Binary: /*noun*/ the concept that only two genders exist and that every person is only either male or female.

Gender Dysphoria: /*noun*/ 1. a medical diagnosis characterized by incongruence between one's experienced and/or expressed gender and assigned gender. 2. the state of feeling uncomfortable with one's body as it relates to assigned gender. 3. the state of being uncomfortable with expectations of gender roles. 4. discomfort with other aspects of gender expression and/or perception, including clothing, makeup, hair style, voice, and so on.

Gender Expression: /*noun*/ outward presentation or expression of gender through dress, appearance, speech patterns, mannerisms, and so on separate from, and sometimes not related to, gender identity. Gender expression may be feminine, masculine, androgynous, or anywhere in between.

Gender Fluid: /*adj.*/ describes a person whose gender identity varies over time or in different circumstances, including male, female, both, neither, or other non-binary identity, or any combination of identities.

Gender Identity: /*noun*/ one's individual, personal sense of being a man, woman, both, neither, or other nonbinary identity. Gender identity is inward and unique to each person, and is separate from outward expression of that identity, or from the perception of that identity by others.

Gender Nonbinary: /*adj.*/ describes a person whose gender identity or expression exists outside the gender binary of exclusively male or exclusively female.

Gender Nonconforming: /*adj.*/ describes a gender presentation or identity that is not aligned with traditional expectations for masculine or feminine and that lies outside the gender binary. Often abbreviated as "GNC."

Gender Normative /*adj.*/ 1. describes a person whose gender expression falls within societal expectations for masculine or feminine.

Gender Perception: /*noun*/ observations and categorizations about gender based on one's perception of another person and how their own gender biases affect the way they move through the world. A person who has strong associations with the gender binary may have a different, more limited sense of gender perception than someone who is not attached to the gender binary.

Gender Policing: /*adj.*/ monitoring or enforcing gender stereotypes, gender roles, or gendered behaviors. Gender policing ranges from discouraging certain gendered behaviors, especially for children, or requiring that someone meet a certain threshold in order to gain acceptance. "For trans or gender-variant people . . . the assumption is that someone is only 'truly' transgender if they have gone through some form of medical and/or surgical transition." (Erickson-Schroth, 2014, p. 614)

Genderqueer: /*adj.*/ describes a person who does not identify within the binary system of male or female; can be used as an umbrella term for other gender nonconforming or nonbinary identities.

Gender Questioning: /*adj.*/ describes a person who is curious about or questioning their own gender identity or is experimenting with gender expression and identity.

Gender Reassignment Surgery (GRS), **Sex Reassignment Surgery** (SRS), **Gender Affirming Surgery:** /*noun*/ surgical options that change a person's external bodily structure from those of one sex to those of another. Surgical options may include gonadoplasty and/or chest reconstruction.

Gender Variant or **Gender Diverse:** /*adj.*/ describes someone whose identity and/or expression does not conform to societal gender norms. This term can be inclusive, but it could be harmful if it is used to imply that these identities are abnormal.

Gynesexual or **Gynephilic:** /*adj.*/ "being primarily sexually, romantically and/or emotionally attracted to some woman, females, and/or femininity" (Killermann, 2017b, p. 264).

Heteronormativity: /*noun*/ the assumption that all people are heterosexual, that heterosexuality is superior to or more natural than other sexualities, and that men should be masculine and women should be feminine.

Heterosexism: /*noun*/ preferential treatment granted to heterosexual or heterosexual-perceived people.

Heterosexual: /*adj.*/ describes a person who is physically, emotionally, and/or romantically attracted to people of the opposite sex/gender.

Homophobia: /*noun*/ 1. the irrational fear or hatred of homosexuals (including bisexuals and transgender individuals), expressed through harmful or violent behavior. 2. **Homophobic:** /*adj.*/ describes an individual who harbors negative attitudes or prejudices towards gay people.

Homosexual: / *adj.* & *noun* / describes someone who is physically, emotionally, and/or romantically attracted to people of the same sex/gender. This term can be harmful, particularly when used as a *noun*, because of its history as a categorization of mental illness.

Hormone Replacement Therapy (HRT): /*noun*/ sometimes used as part of the transition process, the introduction of hormones to the body that align with one's gender identity.

Intersex: /*adj.*/ describes a person whose chromosomes, hormones, and internal or external sex organs differ from traditionally male or female characteristics. Previously known by the term *hermaphrodite* but that term is outdated and derogatory and must not be used.

Lesbian: /*adj.*/ describes someone who identifies as female and is physically, romantically, and sexually attracted to other females.

LGBTQ, **LGBTQIA**, **LGBTQ+**, or other variations: /*abbreviation*/ "shorthand or umbrella terms for all folks who have a non-normative (or queer) gender or sexuality, there are many different initialisms people prefer. There is no "correct" initialism or acronym—what is preferred varies by person, region, and often evolves over time" (Killermann, 2017b, p. 266). LGBTQIA stands for lesbian, gay, bisexual, transgender, queer (or questioning), intersex, asexual.

Masculine-of-Center: /*adj.*/ describes a person whose identity, presentation, or relationships to others reside in the range of masculine but who does not necessarily identify as a man.

Misgender: /*verb*/ to incorrectly presume or identify a person's gender, whether intentionally or unintentionally. Misgendering can happen by using incorrect name or pro*noun*s or making statements or assumptions about one's behavior or presentation based on inaccurate gender perception.

MtF: /*abbreviation*/ stands for "male to female." Mostly used in a medical context and should be avoided because of the implication that a person goes *from* one gender *to* another, rather than having always identified as their affirmed gender.

Mx.: /"mix" or "schwa"/ a gender-neutral honorific that many nonbinary identifying people prefer. *"Mx. Johnson is a caring therapist."*

Neutrois: /*adj.*/ describes someone with a gender-neutral identity who may wish to exhibit a gender-neutral presentation or body.

Outing: /*verb*/ accidental or unwanted disclosure of someone's gender identity or sexual orientation.

Pansexual: /*adj.*/ describes a person who is physically, emotionally, and/or romantically attracted to a person of any sex and/or gender. Sometimes shortened to "pan."

Passing: /*adj. & verb*/ trans people being accepted and/or perceived as their self-identified gender identity without others identifying them as trans.

Preferred Gender Pronouns or **Preferred Pronouns:** /*noun*/ the set of pronouns that an individual would like others to use when talking to or about them.

Queer: /*adj.*/ an umbrella term to describe individuals who do not identify as straight and/or have a non-normative gender identity. It is not accepted by all members of the LGBTQ+ community due to its historically derogatory use.

Questioning: /*adj.*/ describes someone who is unsure or learning more about their sexual orientation or gender identity before identifying as LGBTQ+ or queer.

Sexual Orientation: /*noun*/ "the type of sexual, romantic, emotional/spiritual attraction one has the capacity to feel for some others, generally labeled based on the gender relationship between the person and the people they are attracted to" (Killermann, 2017b, p. 269).

Straight: /*adj.*/ a colloquial term for heterosexual.

Third Gender: /*noun*/ 1. a gender category used by both modern and historic societies that recognize more than two genders. 2. a term used by some people, meaning different things to different people, as a way to progress beyond the gender binary.

Top Surgery: /*noun*/ colloquial term describing chest reconstructive surgery intended to influence gender expression and/or perception to be more masculine or feminine.

Trans: /*abbreviation*/ a shorthand of the word *transgender*. (see "Transgender")

Trans*: /*abbreviation*/ trans with an asterisk is often used in written forms (not spoken) to allow for more inclusivity of all gender identities, including nonbinary identities.

Transgender: /*adj.*/ describes a person whose self-experienced gender is not the same as the gender/sex they were assigned at birth.

Transgender Man, **Trans Man**, or **Transmasculine Individual:** /*noun*/ individual assigned female at birth but who identifies and/or lives as male.

Transgender Woman, **Trans Woman**, or **Transfeminine Individual:** /*noun*/ individual assigned male at birth but who identifies and/or lives as female.

Transition: /*noun*/ the process by which a person alters their appearance or the way they move through the world to be aligned with their gender identity and/or the gender by which they wish to be perceived. Transition is deeply personal and can include social, medical, and/or legal aspects.

Transphobia: /*noun*/ fear, hatred, prejudice, or mistreatment of transgender people.

Transsexual: /*adj.*/ an older and outdated term for "transgender" which originated in the medical and psychological communities.

Two-Spirit /*adj.*/ "refers to a person who has both a masculine and a feminine spirit, and is used by some First Nations people to describe their sexual, gender and/or spiritual identity." (University of Toronto, 2017)

Problematic Terminology

Sometimes, knowing what to say isn't as important as what *not* to say. Most of the time, the communication mistakes we make are unintentional and lack malice, but they can still be hurtful or offensive. The following list contains common, yet easily avoidable, language mistakes. These problematic terms and phrases are often offensive and/or outdated and sometimes grammatically incorrect. Preferred language choices are listed with brief explanations to their logic and rationale.

PROBLEMATIC: "transgenders," "a transgender"

PREFERRED: "transgender people," "a transgender person"

Transgender should be used as an adjective, not a *noun*. Do not say, "Mary is a transgender," or "The performance included many transgenders." Instead say, "Mary is a transgender person," or "The performance included many transgender people."

PROBLEMATIC: "transgendered" or "cisgendered"

PREFERRED: "transgender" or "cisgender"

The words *transgender* and *cisgender* never need the extraneous "-ed" at the end of the word. Only verbs can be transformed into participles by adding "-ed" and since the words *transgender* and *cisgender* are adjectives, adding "-ed" is grammatically incorrect.

PROBLEMATIC: "transgenderism"

PREFERRED: "being transgender" or "trans identity"

Transgender people do not use this term. This term reduces being transgender to an illness or pathology and is used to dehumanize transgender people.

PROBLEMATIC: "sex change," "preoperative," "postoperative"

PREFERRED: "medical transition"

A person does not need to have surgery in order to transition. Using these problematic terms overemphasizes the importance of surgery when discussing the process of transition for transgender people. Each person's transition is personal and unique and may or may not include any medical intervention.

PROBLEMATIC: "biologically male," "biologically female," "genetically male," "genetically female," "born a man," "born a woman"

PREFERRED: "assigned male at birth," "assigned female at birth" or "designated male at birth," "designated female at birth"

These problematic phrases oversimplify very complex aspects of sex and gender. There are as many iterations of biological gender as there are people in the world.

PROBLEMATIC: "passing"

PREFERRED: N/A

Passing is a controversial term because it gives the power to the observer rather than giving full agency to the individual. Some folks place high priority on "passing" while others do not, and having others perceive an individual as having "passed" is not always a positive experience.

PROBLEMATIC: "female to male (FtM)" or "male to female (MtF)"

PREFERRED: "trans male," "transgender man," "trans man," "trans masculine," or "trans female," "transgender woman," "trans woman," "trans feminine"

These terms imply that the individual was once one gender and then changed or switched to the other. Although the individual's birth-assigned sex is listed first, that person likely never identified as that gender. The notion that a trans person changed *from* female *to* male or *from* male *to* female is not correct as this is confusing birth-assigned sex with a person's self-identified gender.

PROBLEMATIC: "hermaphrodite"

PREFERRED: "intersex person"

Hermaphrodite is an outdated term that is sometimes still used to sensationalize intersex people.

PROBLEMATIC: "transsexual"

PREFERRED: "transgender"

Transsexual is mostly considered an outdated term, but there are still some people who prefer the use of that term to describe themselves. Unlike *transgender*, the term *transsexual* is not an umbrella term and many transgender people do not like to be referred to as transsexual.

PROBLEMATIC: "transvestite"

PREFERRED: "cross-dresser"

Transvestite is an outdated term and has some potentially negative connotations.

RECOMMENDED READING

Adams, C. (2017, March 24). *The gender identity terms you need to know*. Retrieved from https://www.cbsnews.com/news/transgender-gender-identity-terms-glossary/

Banis, O. (2012, September 2). *What's my voice type? The different voice types and how to distinguish them*. Retrieved from http://choirly.com/whats-my-voice-type/

Beyond the binary, nonbinary, gender identities, gender fluid. (2015, February 22). Retrieved from http://gender.wikia.com/wiki/Gender_Fluid

Butler, M. P. (2016, March 1). *Improving cultural competence to reduce health disparities*. Rockville, MD: Agency for Healthcare Research and Quality.

Castanho, C. (2017). Gender diversity and education in musical theater. *Huffington Post*. Retrieved from https://www.huffingtonpost.com/entry/gender-diversity-and-education-in-musical-theatre_us_58b62c6ee4b0658fc20f9b81

Check, M. P. (2012, August 26). *Deconstructing cisprivilege and what it means to be trans**. Retrieved from https://cisprivilegecheck.wordpress.com/2012/08/04/terminology-how-to-refer-to-a-trans-person/

Davies, S. (2016, Spring). Training the transgender singer: Finding the voice inside. *Journal of Singing*, pp. 10–11.

Davies, S. V. (2015, November 16). Voice and communication change for gender nonconforming individuals: Giving voice to the person inside. *International Journal of Transgenderism*.

GLAAD. (2017, September 28). *Tips for allies of transgender people*. Retrieved from https://www.glaad.org/transgender/allies

GLAAD media reference guide. (2017, September 24). Retrieved from https://www.glaad.org/reference/transgender

Kilman, C. (2013, Summer). The gender spectrum. *Teaching Tolerance Magazine, 44*.

Kilman, C. (2017, September 30). *Creating a gender-inclusive classroom*. Retrieved from https://www.tolerance.org/magazine/summer-2013/the-gender-spectrum

Know your rights: Transgender people and the law. (2017, September 27). Retrieved from https://www.aclu.org/know-your-rights/transgender-people-and-law

Lesbian, Gay, Bisexual, Transgender Resource Center. (2017, September 15). University of Wisconsin Milwaukee. Retrieved from https://uwm.edu/lgbtrc/support/gender-pronouns/

Newcomer, N. (2004, January 9). *Boys will be girls, girls will be boys: Cross gender roles in opera*. Retrieved from http://library.buffalo.edu/music/exhibits/genderroles.pdf

Nichols, J. (2013, September 20). Rie's story, Ryan's journey: Music in the life of a transgender student. *Journal of Research in Music Education*.

Wilkinson, W. (2014, May 1). Cultural competency. *Transgender Studies Quarterly, 1*(1–2), 68–73.

REFERENCES

Botswick, J. M. & Martin, K. A. (2007). A man's brain in an ambiguous body: A case of mistaken gender identity. *The American Journal of Psychiatry, 164*(10), 1499–1505.

Dragowski, E. A., Scharrón-del Río, M. R., Sandigorsky, A. L. (2011). Childhood gender identity . . . disorder? Developmental, cultural, and diagnostic concerns. *Journal of Counseling & Development, 89*, 360–366.

Erickson-Schroth, L. (Ed.). (2014). *Trans bodies, trans selves: A resource for the transgender community.* New York, NY: Oxford University Press.

Gilbert, S. F. (2000) Chromosomal sex determination in mammals. In S. F. Gilbert (Ed.), *Developmental Biology* (6th ed.). Sunderland, MA: Sinauer Associates. Retrieved from https://www.ncbi.nlm.nih.gov/books/NBK9967/

Jones, Laci. (2009). The third sex: Gender identity development of intersex persons. *Graduate Journal of Counseling Psychology, 1*(2), 1–9.

Killermann, S. (2017a). *The genderbread person.* Retrieved from http://itspronouncedmetrosexual.com/2015/03/the-genderbread-person-v3/#sthash.v8KHvrwW.dpbs

Killermann, S. (2017b). *A guide to gender: The social justice advocate's handbook.* Austin, TX: Impetus Books.

Kranz, G.S., Hahn, A., Kaufmann, U., Külblöck, M., Hummer, A., Ganger, S., . . . Lanzenberger, R. (2014, November). White matter microstructure in transsexuals and controls investigated by diffusion tensor imaging. *The Journal of Neuroscience, 34*(46), 15466–15475.

The Trevor Project. (2013, January 20). *LGBTQ terminology.* Philadelphia, PA.

University of Toronto. (2017). *Two-spirit community.* Retrieved from http://lgbtqhealth.ca/community/two-spirit.php

CHAPTER
2

Communication

I'm one of those people who, from earliest memory, always felt feminine-identified even though I was assigned male at birth . . . I didn't have a good explanation for those feelings when I was younger . . . I know only that those feelings persist no matter what. I know that they make me who I am to myself, whatever other people may feel about me or do toward me for having them.

—Susan Stryker, *Transgender History: The Roots of Today's Revolution* (p. X)

INTRODUCTION

Clear and compassionate communication are cornerstones of effective work for voice training professions. Most voice training is either individual or in small groups, resulting in close and meaningful student-teacher relationships. Voice teachers can become mentors and confidants to students, nurturing their success as singers and dynamic human beings, creating bonds through mutual respect. The voice studio can be a safe haven for students to explore identity and artistry if the teacher has set parameters to encourage that freedom. This chapter contains suggestions for reevaluating and reorganizing communication in a gender-inclusive studio or institution, to ensure that all students feel welcome, supported, respected, and safe.

GENDER INCLUSIVITY IN THE CLASSROOM AND STUDIO

A student's success depends on feeling comfortable in their learning environment, and especially for transgender students, an affirming and gender-inclusive classroom is a must in order to allow creativity and artistic growth. If the atmosphere is uncertain, the student will most likely feel unsafe to experiment, make mistakes, and truly express themselves. Carving out and maintaining a gender-inclusive studio or classroom involves self-reflection of personal gender experience, awareness and dissolution of gender biases, creating boundaries that give room for students to flourish, and setting examples of gender-conscious behavior through daily interactions and reevaluation of potentially harmful or exclusive language. The process is no small feat, but the rewards are great.

Gender inclusivity and affirmation of others first begins with internal reflection, self-awareness, and self-acceptance. Teachers who are truly fellow travelers with their transgender and gender nonbinary students will walk the path of gender exploration alongside them by asking, "What is *my* gender? How do I express my gender with my voice?" Acknowledging and naming the ways in which the voice expresses gender, especially for the teacher, opens avenues for discussion and reflection. There may be instances when the teacher inadvertently performs or expects students to perform gender stereotypes through vocal demonstration or explanation of technique. While such demonstrations can be helpful, cognizance of the performative nature of gender, especially as vocal artists, should be forefront on the mind of the teacher. Maintain awareness during moments when the student experiences even subtle discomfort by developing familiarity and common understanding about the myriad ways dysphoria manifests, and practice empathy and compassion for students who are navigating those challenges. To build bridges toward effective communication, teachers must first evaluate and express their own experiences of gender and voice.

The next step of the teacher's journey into understanding gender is developing awareness of their own interactions with the world through the lens of gender. Take a self-inventory of obstacles and limitations that gender norms and stereotypes present, or judgments and beliefs about gender that may limit the ability to develop empathy, or limit the student's freedom of expression in the studio. Associations and expectations about voice and gender may be deep-rooted and difficult to discard, and it may be disorienting to practice new pronouns, names, or gender-inclusive language for students in transition, but the responsibility to continue to work toward cultural competence lies first with teacher. Notice when automatic or subconscious assumptions arise about someone's gender identity and quiet those assumptions.

During the process of self-reflection, interactions with students will likely begin to shift, and practicing healthy boundaries with students is crucial to their safety and growth. Students will reveal their own story in their own time, and there may be aspects about transition or trans identity that, despite the teacher's curiosity, have nothing to do with the student's voice training. Genuine and compassionate interest in the student's artistic goals and progress helps create a space where the student can freely share. If a student is open to discussing their own gender identity, believe and affirm them without hesitation or qualifiers. There are no thresholds to being "trans enough," and someone's gender identity is dependent only on how they experience themselves; trans or nonbinary identity is not dependent on surgeries, hormones, or other aspects of transition. Similarly, gender identity is not static; it fluctuates and evolves. Give room for the student to share new thoughts or revelations about their gender and continually uncover the ways in which voice is, or is not, an integral part of their gender expression.

Although it is necessary to discuss differences in training for transgender singers in the context of this text, reducing trans singers to only their gender identity is harmful and unhelpful. Each student has a spectrum of interests, talents, thoughts, and experiences, which may or may not be related to gender, that make up their whole personality. Often trans students are unwittingly presented with the burden of educating their own teachers on gender theory, trans issues, and transition. Search out resources and guidance on these topics so that the student can focus on their own journey, supported by a well-informed and knowledgeable teacher.

Through self-reflection and self-affirmation of one's own gender identity and expression, teachers can begin to show that affirmation outwardly toward others. As an example, interactions with students and colleagues set the tone for a gender-inclusive space by utilizing introductions that include preferred pronouns. During the first class of the semester, a teacher may begin by saying, "Hello everyone! Welcome to our first class of the semester. My name is Professor Kay Jones and my pronouns are she/her," and then going on to ask students to introduce themselves with their preferred names and pronouns as well. A word of caution, however. This exercise is counterproductive if asking students to state their pronouns could single out a gender-diverse person. If a trans/nonbinary student has already come out, it is appropriate to ask that student permission to encourage their classmates to practice introductions with pronouns in this way. Shifting the paradigm away from cisnormativity benefits everyone in the room.

Introductions that give room for gender affirmation can initiate gender-inclusive communication; maintaining that communication involves reevaluating and carefully selecting gender-neutral language in the classroom and studio. Classroom settings are among the heavily gendered environments that students must navigate throughout the course of their voice education. Culturally competent communication requires awareness of cisnormativity in traditionally gender binary spaces such as choruses and rehearsals as well, where shifting language is helpful. Instead of asking for "all the men," use gender-neutral language such as "low voices" or "basses and tenors." There may be a low-voiced singer who does not identify as a man who will be excluded by gendered language, and choosing accurate descriptors of voice parts, rather than short-cutting to gendered language, will likely lead to more effective rehearsals regardless of the gender makeup of the ensemble. Bathrooms and dressing rooms can be gendered as well. Allow students to utilize the facilities in which they are most comfortable and, if possible, create gender neutral spaces or all-gender spaces for those facilities. This will help support the safety of the students and establish a consistent expectation among fellow students and colleagues that gender identity will be honored and respected.

Box 2–1. Gender Self-Reflection Worksheet for Teachers

1. What is my gender? _____

2. Which pronouns do I prefer? _____

3. What obstacles or limitations have I faced due to either my gender identity, gender expression, or how others perceive my gender?

   _____

   _____

4. In what ways do I express my gender with my voice?

   _____

   _____

5. What are some of the things that I notice about a person that lead me to make assumptions about their gender (whether intentionally or not)?

   _____

   _____

6. What judgments do I have about gender? (Try to be honest, without self-judgement for having judgments.)

   _____

   _____

7. What can I do to reevaluate and reconsider those judgments to be more gender inclusive and affirming?

   _____

   _____

8. How can I start creating a gender-inclusive environment by presenting a positive model?

   Example:

   Hi, my name is _____ and my

   pronouns are _____.

   _____

   _____

Insidious Gendered Language

In English, nouns do not have a grammatical gender as other languages do. In French, *le* is the definite article for masculine nouns and *la* is the definite article for feminine nouns. Gendered nouns are common in other languages, but in English there is no equivalent. One would say *the pen* or *the house*, using the same genderless definite article *the* for both. There are, however, words, phrases, idioms, and colloquialisms in English that unnecessarily impose gender in the language. Often the intent is innocuous and without malice, but the use of it can lead to a transgender student feeling excluded or invisible.

Examples of gender-exclusive language include phrases that assume a binary system of gender and/or assume all people are male-identified: "boys and girls," "ladies and gentlemen," "his or her," "brothers and sisters," "you guys," "mankind," "all men are created equal," and so on. Gender-inclusive language assumes there are identities that fall between or outside the gender binary and strive to leave no one out: "honored guests," "siblings," "everyone," "human kind," and so on. Table 2–1 demonstrates examples of terms and phrases commonly used in the classroom. The left side lists the gendered version and the right side lists the recommended gender-neutral adjustment.

Although these shifts in language may seem insignificant, for a trans or nonbinary person, they are substantial and deeply meaningful. Gendered language excludes and in some cases completely erases gender-diverse people, and creating a paradigm of culturally competent communication relies on acknowledgment and celebration of gender diversity. Practic-

Table 2–1. Terms and Phrases Commonly Used in the Classroom

Gendered Version	Gender-Neutral Version
"Let's have all the *women* sing the top line in measures 46 to 59."	"Let's have all the *altos and sopranos* sing the top line in measures 46 to 59."
"*Ladies and gentlemen*, please turn to page 6."	"*Everyone*, please turn to page 6."
"Each person selects *his or her* own research topic."	"Each person selects *their* own research topic."
"This song cycle is written for *male* singers."	"This song cycle is written for *voices with a range of G2 to E4*."

ing gender-inclusive language communicates to the student that they are seen and that the teacher is actively working to build a safe, nourishing environment for them to learn.

Preferred Name

Some transgender people choose to change their name as part of social or legal transition to find a name that better aligns with their own self-experience. In the article "Why It's So Important to Respect Transgender People's Chosen Names," Lore-Graham (2016) writes,

> The act of choosing a name is an empowering one. It is redefining a core aspect of one's self, what one is called and how one is identified to the world, in accordance with one's own identity. For transgender people, for example, picking a new name allows one to choose an identifier that fits with one's desired gender and presentation. For others, it might signal a new stage in one's life. (para. 8)

Choosing a name is a deeply personal aspect of transition, as are all parts of transition. If a student asks to be called by a new preferred name, respect and do so without debate or resistance. Calling someone by their birth name, or *dead name*, after having changed it—whether the legal procedures for name change have been completed or not—is called *dead-naming* and is harmful. There may be instances where knowledge of the previous name of an individual is necessary for documentation, and in those cases, using the phrase "legal name" or "given name" is much less harmful than requesting someone's "real name." Any time a student is forced to list or be referred to by their dead name, it can be a significant source of dysphoria and discomfort. During auditions, intake, or entrance procedures, including an option for preferred name gives the student agency over how they are called by teachers and others within the institution. Once a student has requested to update their preferred name, make concerted efforts to use that name consistently. During conversations with the student about their preferred name, discuss when and with whom it is appropriate to use that name and if there are scenarios in which the student needs to be referred to by their given name. For example, they may ask to be referred to by their preferred name in the studio but by their given name with their parents if they have not yet come out to their family. Give room for the student to claim agency and autonomy about how they are recognized by teachers, fellow students, administrators, and others in their social environments.

Pronouns

Third-person pronouns refer to people in place of proper nouns or names. For example, "Adam went to the store" becomes "he went to the store," if Adam prefers he/him pronouns. Table 2–2 shows a somewhat comprehensive, but not complete, list of pronouns and their usage.

It is important not to make assumptions about an individual's pronouns based on their appearance or physical characteristics, and it is always best to use gender-neutral language or refer to someone by their name until there is opportunity to ask about preferred pronouns. As discussed in Chapter 1, a person's gender expression may or may not be congruent with the gender norms of a particular society, and immediate or automatic associations or judgments based on initial perception may be inaccurate or in some cases harmful. Although it can feel awkward at first, it is certainly appropriate to ask, "What pronouns do you prefer?" Or, "Will you remind me again of your pronouns?"

Table 2–2. Common Pronouns and Usage

She is singing	I just saw her	Her bag is there	This is hers	She did it herself
She	Her	Her	Hers	Herself
He	Him	His	His	Himself
They	Them	Their	Theirs	Themselves
Zie	Zim	Zir	Zis	Zieself
Sie	Sie	Hir	Hirs	Hirself
Ey	Em	Eir	Eirs	Eirself
Ve	Ver	Vis	Vers	Verself
Tey	Ter	Tem	Ters	Terself
E	Em	Eir	Eirs	Emself

Box 2–2. Robin's Pronouns

1. When referring to Robin, whose pronouns are he/him/his:

   "*He* borrowed my music book, and I returned *his*. *His* lesson today was terrific! I'm proud of *him*."

2. When referring to Robin, whose pronouns are she/her/hers:

   "*She* borrowed my music book, and I returned *hers*. *Her* lesson today was terrific! I'm proud of *her*."

3. When referring to Robin, whose pronouns are they/them/theirs:

   "*They* borrowed my music book, and I returned *theirs*. *Their* lesson today was terrific! I'm proud of *them*."

4. When referring to Robin, about whom preferred pronouns have not been stated:

   "*Robin* borrowed my music book, and I returned *Robin's*. *Robin's* lesson today was terrific! I'm proud of *Robin*."

Mistakes Happen

Navigating the nuanced and colorful realm of gender may be a new experience for some teachers, and mistakes are only natural. Even within transgender communities, peers, colleagues, and friends accidentally misgender or dead name others, and acknowledge the learning process with compassion and patience. Often, mistakes are not made out of malice or ill intention, but a simple slip is easier to forgive than a mistake made out of willful ignorance. When well-meaning mistakes arise, it is appropriate to apologize, make the correction, and move on. It is inappropriate to dwell on and belabor the mistake, forcing the person about whom the mistake was made to take emotional care of their conversation partner. It is also inappropriate to become defensive or resistant to making the correction or to claim grammatical correctness in situations where grammar is unrelated to the situation at hand. Avoiding situations for fear of offending someone else or fear of making the mistake is also unhelpful and stagnates movement toward gender-inclusive communication.

The realm of voice education can be fraught with insecurity, fueled by competition, reinforced by performance expectations. It is only natural to feel compelled to support students in transition through such stress, and open communication achieves that. Remarking on appearance or making attempts to affirm a trans or nonbinary person in a way that reduces them to gender may be less helpful. The backhanded compliment or helpful tip is a common yet easily avoidable mistake. Avoid these examples below, which may be well intentioned but are extremely hurtful:

"I would have never known you were transgender."

"He looks exactly like a real man."

"She's so beautiful. I would have never guessed she was transgender."

"He's so good looking. Even though he's transgender, I'd date him."

"Being transgender must be so hard. You're so brave."

"You'd look more like a girl if you wore less makeup."

Instead, try:

"How do you feel about your voice today?"

"What can I do to support you?"

"What would make you feel comfortable and confident going into this audition?"

"How would it feel to embody this male/female/gender-neutral character?"

SAFEKEEPING SOMEONE'S TRANSGENDER IDENTITY

Transgender people are persecuted and ostracized in communities all over the world. Physical safety for trans people is difficult to find, and emotional safety even more so. The voice studio provides emotional and artistic safety for students throughout their vocal journey and should be a safe place for trans and nonbinary students as well. When a student shares their feelings about gender or details about their identity or transition, it is important to keep that information secure until the student decides to make it public in their own way. Unless given specific permission to share information about a student's identity, do not impart that information to anyone else, or leave opportunity for it to be disseminated accidentally. Some of the possible repercussions of outing a student could be loss of friends, getting fired from their job, being ostracized in their community, or even physical harm.

In a 2014 article in *The Washington Post*, Rich Ferraro of the Gay and Lesbian Alliance Against Discrimination states,

> It is never appropriate to disclose the fact that someone is transgender without [their] explicit permission. We live in a culture that marginalizes transgender people, subjecting them to poverty, discrimination and violence—and outing them places them in actual physical danger. A person should be allowed to make [their] own decision about facing the consequences of being an out transgender person. Transgender people are simply living their lives like everyone else—and they deserve the same respect and privacy accorded other people. (Fahri, 2014, para. 5)

Outing a student is likely unintentional, and awareness of the possible scenarios in which a student is exposed prevents accidentally sharing private information. Be mindful of conversation topics and content, surroundings, and potential listeners.

Box 2–3. Alex

Alex unfortunately suffered as an example of what not to do. Alex is a trans man who had been taking lessons only for a short time. As his lesson came to a close, the next student walked into the studio, and the two were introduced. Final thoughts about Alex's lesson were discussed as the next student was unpacking and getting ready to begin.

At the start of his next lesson, Alex expressed deep concern about his personal information being exposed to others, which was alarming and disconcerting. He explained that because there was another student in the room, it was extremely inappropriate to continue talking about his voice at that point. Part of the discussion was about Alex's hormone treatment and the effects it was having on his voice. Alex had been accidentally, but very obviously, outed in that conversation. It was a horrendous mistake that will never happen again.

It is easy to take for granted simple interactions with students such as making lesson plans, sending emails, or even greeting students in the hallway or on the street. Protecting someone's trans identity, however, requires careful thought about the gravity and implication that those interactions can have. Even if a transgender or nonbinary student has shared that part of their identity, it does not mean they are ready to share it with the rest of the world, or even the rest of the department. Utilize the following questions to gain clarity about the safest ways to communicate with the student while they are outside the lesson studio.

1. *Which name would you like me to use in formal communication?*
   The name your student uses with you in lessons may be the same or different from the name they use with others. As a result, if communication is intercepted or overheard, it may accidentally expose the student.

2. *How would you like me to contact you with lesson/class information?*
   Some students may not want the fact that they are training their voice to be public knowledge. This is especially true for teachers/voice professionals specializing in speech masculinization or feminization.

3. *If I see you in the hall, or even on the street, is it OK if I say hello, and if so, how would you like me to address you?*
   There may still be parts of a student's life that are not public knowledge and they may use a different name or pronouns, dress differently, or behave differently in other social scenarios or situations. Talking with them in that state may also cause a great deal of anxiety and dysphoria, in addition to potentially exposing parts of themselves that are not public.

4. *Which name and pronouns would you like me to use when talking with your family?*
   This is especially important for young students who may not have revealed their transgender identity to their family or who need someone in their corner to demonstrate correct usage of their name and pronouns. The name and/or pronouns they prefer may be the same or different from how their family refers to them. A simple mistake here could accidentally out a student.

5. *How would you like me to list you in the performance program?*

When preparing a performance program, it is wise to assume that the student has not come out to everyone who will be in attendance. Make sure to find out how they feel most comfortable being listed in the program.

STUDENT HISTORY

When a student starts voice lessons with a new teacher, it is common practice to gather historical information such as previous vocal training, performance experience, and vocal health. This is welcomed and necessary as it helps teachers design a successful path for the voice student. When training a transgender singer, most of the needed historical information is identical to that of a cisgender student, with some consideration for aspects of transition that pertain to vocal training. Figure 2–1 shows a sample student history form that includes questions relevant to vocal transition.

Questions pertaining specifically to aspects of transition that affect voice include hormone therapy, body-shaping garments, surgeries, and specific goals or challenges around vocal dysphoria. Preceding questions about preferred name, pronouns, and method of contact are useful for all new students, regardless of identity, in the context of a gender-inclusive studio. As explained previously, careful consideration about communication through email or phone ensures the student's safety.

Chapters 5 and 6 offer detailed information about body-shaping garments and hormone therapy and their effects on voice. Knowledgeable and open discussion about these aspects of medical transition equip the student to take ownership of their vocal goals and may ease some stress about the qualifications of their new teacher. In addition to familiarity with aspects of social and medical transition, effective communication also requires compassion and care, to ensure that the student is fully seen and heard and never dehumanized or treated as a special case in need of accommodation.

During new student intake, teachers can also inquire into how the student feels about the sound of their voice. This may be a new or unusual question for some teachers, but it is an important consideration when developing a successful pedagogical plan. Some transgender singers want to change the timbre and range of their voice; others do not. For some, voice is a source of dysphoria and the sound of their voice does not reflect how they would like to express themselves. Others are content and have no interest in drastically changing

NEW STUDENT INFORMATION SHEET

Student Name: _____

Pronouns: _____

Address: _____ Apt: _____

    City: _____ State: _____ Zip: _____

Phone: _____ Email: _____

Preferred method of contact: _____

Would you like to be added to the mailing list? YES   NO

VOICE HISTORY INFORMATION

Are you currently on any hormone therapy treatment? _____
If yes, please describe type(s), dosage, frequency, and length of treatment:

_____

Have you had any operations that would affect your voice? (tracheal shave, FFS, VFS, etc.)?

_____

Have you ever taken voice lessons or received voice training?   YES   NO
If yes, please describe:

_____

Have you ever had problems with your voice? i.e. chronic hoarseness, sore throat, long periods of laryngitis, hemorrhage, nodules, cysts, polyps, or other lesions.

YES   NO   If yes, please describe:

_____

Do you smoke?   YES   NO

What are your goals for voice training?

_____

Figure 2–1. Sample Student Intake Form.

the quality of the voice but are looking for guidance to improve technique or explore new artistic avenues. Open and flexible goals give the student support and autonomy throughout their voice training. Student-led voice education may be a new experience for some teachers, but the satisfaction that both student and teacher share upon reaching the student's goals is exciting and motivating.

Just as there are aspects of a person's transition that pertain to vocal training, other historical information does not. Asking about transgender identity, transgender communities, gender reassignment surgery, or other aspects of transition that are in no way related to voice is invasive and places a heavy and undue burden on the student. Although the student is an expert in their own gender and voice experience, it is unfair to expect them to be an expert in all aspects of trans identity. Students offer opportunities for teachers to learn but cannot bear the responsibility of educating their educators about gender identity.

SUCCESSFUL COMMUNICATION

Gender-conscious communication involves compassion, knowledge, experience, patience, and a willingness to take risks. Introducing oneself with pronouns for the first time might be unnerving but is a necessary first step to normalizing gender-diverse identities. Having open discussions about goals and allowing the student to lead the vocal journey is a worthwhile endeavor that benefits everyone. Compassionate curiosity about each student's experience of their own voice opens opportunities for truly authentic expression, freedom, and confidence as a singer. Make room to challenge deeply rooted beliefs about gender identity and expression, uphold expectations that all gender identities deserve respect and support, and students will flourish in the voice studio and beyond.

REFERENCES

Fahri, Paul. (2014). Grantland offers two sides on divisive article about transgender inventor who killed herself. *The Washington Post*. Retrieved from https://www.washingtonpost.com/lifestyle/style/grantland-offers-two-sides-on-divisive-article-about-transgender-inventor-who-killed-herself/2014/01/21/492f8162-82aa-11e3-8099-9181471f7aaf_story.html?utm_term=.64a93aa3c0b1

Lore-Graham. (2016, February 9). *Why it's so important to respect transgender people's chosen names*. Retrieved from https://www.xojane.com/issues/transgender-names

Stryker, Susan. (2008). *Transgender history: The roots of today's revolution*. New York, NY: Seal Press.

Voice Classification and Repertoire

The possibility missed by. . . various popular media is this: the culture may not simply be creating roles for naturally gendered people, the culture may in fact be <u>creating</u> the gendered people.

—Kate Bornstein, *Gender Outlaw: On Men, Women, and the Rest of Us* (pp. 14–15)

INTRODUCTION

Gender and voice have long been linked together in music training and the music business. Programs and institutions factor in gender when designing a training regimen for voice students, determining voice type, and assigning repertoire. Professional and preprofessional organizations such as universities, performance ensembles, and casting agencies heavily consider gender when determining acceptance and casting. There are certain vocal sounds, inflections, and speech patterns that are sometimes perceived as feminine or masculine, and those traits influence the way teachers hear and guide singers. This chapter raises questions about the influence of gender on voice categorization, repertoire selection, and casting, to encourage singing teachers to deconstruct some of the gender binaries that can limit singing students.

SOUNDING MASCULINE, SOUNDING FEMININE

Labeling a voice as masculine or feminine is problematic in the gender-inclusive voice studio, because it ties the quality of the voice to the gender identity of the singer. A male-identified person with a high range and light timbre is no more or less of a man than a singer with a low voice range and dark timbre. A female-identified person with a low voice range who sings traditional baritone repertoire does not have a "masculine" voice any more than a female-identified soprano, because they both identify as women; the femininity of both singers is not intrinsically linked to their voices, and neither voice has intrinsically gendered characteristics. Any associations that have been made between voice range, voice quality, and gender were created out of an outdated necessity to maintain the gender binary. Gender-conscious voice teachers can provide a more inclusive studio by removing those associations and allowing space for a person's gender identity to exist alongside their singing identity, rather than being tied to it.

When guiding singers toward their voice goals, it is important to choose careful language. Try using specific adjectives to describe the desired sound rather than any associations with gender. Words like broader, lower, chestier, darker, deeper, lighter, floatier, headier, loftier, and so on can guide the student toward a different production without bringing any discussion of gendered voice into the education process. Anatomically and functionally accurate terminology is another effective substitute.

IDENTIFYING VOICE TYPE

The assignment of voice types and repertoire in a gender-inclusive studio can be a confusing area for many teachers. Gender binary systems have dictated singing parts and voice types for centuries, and reimagining the way we hear and categorize voices can feel daunting. Historically, low-range voice part labels (bass, baritone, tenor) are reserved for men, and high-range voice part labels (alto, mezzo-soprano, soprano) are for women. Even voices that sing some of the same repertoire and have similar qualities have different voice types for different genders, like in the case of counter tenors, contraltos, and some mezzo-sopranos. Upcoming generations of students are less and less tied to gender binaries, including those associated with voice type, but the idea that men can be sopranos and women can be basses is still met with resistance by some of the singing teaching community.

Several factors help singing teachers delineate voice categories and guide students toward repertoire and roles. Vocal range, tessitura, timbre, weight, and location of passaggi all influence how we might label a voice, in addition to the convenient label of gender. But why do we take the gender of the singer into account when we classify voices? Does the singer's gender identity somehow change the sound of their singing voice?

Table 3–1 lists average ranges and the traditional gender assignments of voice types as listed in *The New Harvard Dictionary of Music* (Randel, 1986). It is interesting to note the amount of overlap in voice range between countertenor and contralto, and yet perhaps the only delineation between the

Table 3–1. Voice Parts and Average Voice Ranges

Voice Type	Range	Gender
Soprano	C4–A5	Female
Mezzo-Soprano	A3–F5	Female
Contralto	F3–D5	Female
Countertenor	G3–D5	Male
Tenor	B2–G4	Male
Baritone	G2–E4	Male
Bass	E2–C4	Male

two is the gender of singer. The table also becomes less useful if a singer demonstrates characteristics of a baritone voice in range and weight, but the singer identifies as female. That voice type currently has no label within the framework of this system. Furthermore, nonbinary singers could demonstrate any number of characteristic traits of a particular voice type but don't fit into the current categorization system.

The systems that are in place in the industry today cannot support gender-diverse singers, and it may be time for this to change. A person's gender identity does not alter the quality and range of their singing voice, unless that person chooses to do so through the process of their transition. Perhaps it is time to reimagine a voice classification system that does not delineate genders and to do away with gender-dependent voice categories. Future researchers in training trans and nonbinary singers will be charged with helping to create this reimagined voice classification system.

REPERTOIRE

Just as with any student, there are some factors to consider in searching for repertoire when working with a trans singer. Beyond the obvious elements such as range, tessitura, musical style, and pedagogical purpose, some factors of repertoire selection directly collide with gender identity. Because the singing instrument is the only instrument that creates words, singers are tasked with telling understandable and compelling stories, either as themselves or through character interpretation. The gender identity of the singer may prove to be a factor when deciding if a piece is the right fit, so that the artistic intent of the singer complements the artistic intent of the composer or librettist.

Universal Versus Plot-Specific Lyrics and Libretto

When analyzing the text of a piece, consider the following two types of lyric: universal and plot specific. A universal lyric has no predetermined context, or can be taken directly out of context without disturbing the cohesion of the story. For example, "Early in the Morning" by Ned Rorem has a universal lyric. The piece does not dictate a preset fictional or nonfictional character and the moments in the story before and after the piece are not established. A plot-specific lyric is one that has a preestablished context or character. These usually come from an opera, musical, or other form of vocal work with a libretto.

Many plot-specific lyrics can be performed as universal lyrics, but it could prove detrimental if the piece is associated with an iconic character or experience. An example of this is the song "Maria" from *West Side Story*. Although the actual lyric could be taken out of context and the song could be about any person named Maria, the characters of Tony and Maria are iconic and directly linked with the performance of the musical and this piece within it. This does not necessarily mean it could never be taken out of context, but it is a factor worth considering.

Opera

The historical realm of opera has included problematic themes surrounding race, class, religion, and gender, but the art form is so beautiful and so revered that we are driven to continue producing it. Modern theaters attempt to reimagine traditional opera repertoire and use more socially conscious practices, aware of the responsibility to contextualize centuries-old stories for 21st-century audiences. Redesigning traditional opera roles to remove heteronormative tendencies in casting and production provides opportunities for diversity and growth. Fringe and new opera is also emerging as a medium to explore new themes and support upcoming artists, including transgender and nonbinary composers and performers.

Box 3–1. Lucia Lucas

Lucia is a professional operatic baritone performing internationally in opera houses and through independent projects. She says that after having learned to "perform" as a male for 30 years, her confidence and competency in performing male roles remains secure as long as she is not required to play that part offstage. She says,

"Transitions are front-loaded, meaning the most difficult times are in the beginning. At first, there may be a temptation for singers to reject roles of their gender assigned at birth, but the farther away they get from the moment of coming out, the easier it is for the characters to be simply a character and not a blueprint for future life.

I would always get upset when I had to play old men, but now I have taken steps to ensure that is not my life path so it doesn't bother me anymore. I recently had to prove to an opera house that I could still play a man. While it seemed silly, it also meant that they took my identity very seriously.

"I would encourage your students to make their own opportunities, especially trans students who feel most comfortable doing things that are not inherently baked into the curriculum. I did my first Marcello in a church very sparsely sold with a conductor who was only 20 years old at the time. We got a bunch of people together who wanted to get extra stuff on their resume. The next time an opportunity came up to do Marcello, it was for a 1,000+-seat opera house. That conductor is also now world famous.

"This is even more important for singers who may feel left out because they don't fit the mold. Changing the genders, singing in different keys, and reimagining roles are all things best tried out in less risky situations. If a trans person wants to try to build a career in opera, they do need the mainstream roles, because side projects can't pay the rent. At this moment, it is not possible to have a career unless you are willing to do drab/drag.

"I'd say in a private situation, let the students work on head voice or chest voice if they want. Let trans girls whose voices have dropped know that you can train their head voice, but it will take a lot of work to get it to be professional grade. Schools are tricky because you have a lesson plan and can't deviate too far from it with recitals and juries each having specific requirements.

"The mainstream opera world is not waiting with open arms for trans/nonbinary singers. They are scared their donors won't approve. We must challenge them and hope for steady progress." (Lucas, 2017)

As singing teachers in private studios and institutions, there is a unique opportunity to challenge the mainstream opera world and to support students as they do the same. Talk with students about the kinds of roles they are passionate about and why, and create room for flexibility in how those roles are performed. Some students may feel comfortable performing roles that align with their personality, regardless of range and tessitura. Perhaps that role can be transposed or altered. It is important to keep in mind that trans people avoid scenarios that might feel inauthentic or overtly contrived; some trans masculine singers feel comfortable in pants roles, and some worry about portraying a false representation as a woman in men's clothing. Continual and open conversations with students, institutions, other singing teachers, and directors is imperative in paving the way for gender-diverse opera singers.

Music Theater

Much like opera, traditional music theater is mired in gender stereotypes and expectations, although more modern works challenge those norms and make room for greater diversity of roles and stories. One such example of a gender-liberated music theater role is the Leading Player from Stephen Schwartz's *Pippin*, who is listed in the character breakdown as "either gender" (Stage Agent, 2017b) or "both" (Music Theatre International, 2017). Although this language implies binary gender, this role could conceivably be played as masculine, feminine, androgynous, or anything in between. The allegory of *Pippin* is universal; there is nothing inherently gendered in this character's archetype and audience members can connect to the story regardless of the actor's gender.

The role of St. Jimmy in the Green Day musical, *American Idiot*, is listed in the character breakdown as "male," but it has enjoyed a gender-variant casting history (Stage Agent, 2017a). Originally performed by actor Tony Vincent, Green Day lead singer Billy Joe Armstrong and rock star Melissa Etheridge also played the role on Broadway (Futterman, 2011). In a 2015 Immersive Warehouse production of *American Idiot* in Los Angeles, St. Jimmy was played by Caitlin Ary (American Idiot LA, 2015).

When casting transgender and/or nonbinary performers, it may be tempting to look to cross-dressing roles such as Albin/ZaZa in *La Cage aux Folles*, Lola/Simon in *Kinky Boots*, or Edna Turnblad in *Hairspray*. Proceed with caution. As with opera, some transgender performers may feel comfortable in these roles while others may not. This determination requires an open and honest dialogue with the actor. Look beyond traditional gender assignments of musical theater roles to determine whether flexibility with the character's gender will significantly alter the story. The challenge emerges when casting directors search for leading roles and ingénues with limited visions of the character.

In a recent article, actress and transgender activist Shakina Nayfack discussed gender-specific casting and means toward reducing hetero- and cisnormativity. She says,

> I think the reason writers create gender-specific characters is the same reason they create racially-specific or age-specific characters: There is an experience and a history that the writer is hoping to capture, an experience and a history that is part of the larger story they are telling. That said, if we're talking about smaller roles that don't require specific experiences or histories to contribute to the storytelling, then yeah, why not say "this role is open to anyone who is quick witted and snarky" for example, or "we need someone grounded and wise," then let the actors do their work to bring those qualities, as opposed to using gender or racial identity as the marker. (Castanho, 2017, para. 20)

Art Song

The rich and varied music within the art song repertory provides myriad opportunities for artistic exploration without attachment to gender and encourages some flexibility for transposition of keys and slight modification of texts. When searching out art song repertoire, students may gravitate toward themes of transformation or transfiguration, celebration of the natural world, love (romantic or otherwise), whimsy, or historical stories. All of these themes are easily found within art song, and much of the music contains universal texts rather than plot specific. Allow students to take part in decisions about art song repertoire and to explore voice ranges that feel natural and authentic within this realm.

Jazz, Pop, Rock, and Other Contemporary Commercial Music

Contemporary commercial music allows for the most freedom and flexibility in transposing keys, changing pronouns within lyrics, and exploring different voice qualities. Context and personality should be considered when choosing songs within this repertoire, along with pedagogical purpose, voice range, and technical requirements.

Performance Traditions

In addition to consideration for appropriate genre when selecting repertoire, it is important to consider pieces that have preestablished performance traditions. Although it may seem like a limiting factor, because many large works and solo pieces have long-established norms for the types of singers and actors who perform them, performance traditions have proven over time to be fluid. Broadway revivals demonstrate fluidity by reimagining and casting traditional roles in ways that better reflect current social climates and priorities. This is the nature of performance traditions; as the population changes and people progress, roles and performance styles mirror that change. It is important when selecting repertoire that we challenge ourselves, breaking away from some of the limitations of tradition to help move the field forward.

COMPETITIONS AND CHORAL CONSIDERATIONS

It is commonplace to use gender categories to establish guidelines for competitions and vocal groups. Separating voices along gender lines limits educational opportunities for some singers, because the use of these categories does not describe all people, and strictly binary categories exclude some singers. A choir listed as "all male" or a competition of "female voices" eliminates or at least confuses whether individuals with other gender identities are allowed to participate, even if their vocal range and quality fit into the choir or competition's parameters. A singer whose voice has the properties of a bass, but who does not identify as male, might not wish to participate in a men's choir but likely would not fit in a women's or treble choir either.

The emergence of transgender choruses presents an exciting opportunity to learn about holding gender-inclusive spaces for groups of singers in such a context. Some choruses, like Resonate Trans Choir in Chicago, have replaced the traditional voice parts of soprano, alto, tenor, and bass with Part I, Part II, Part III, and Part IV. Singers in the chorus have the option to choose a voice part based on their comfort level with the range and tessitura of that part. These singers also openly discuss gender associations with different voice parts and any dysphoria that arises from singing in a high or low range. Participants explore different parts of their voice and find relief from vocal dysphoria through freedom to sing a voice part that may not have been available to them in other ensembles. Unique arrangements of choral pieces also support trans and nonbinary singers in order to discover which ranges and musical styles feel the most natural and authentic, and priority is given to trans and nonbinary choral composers.

Gender-inclusive choirs do not need to be special cases, however. It might benefit trans communities even more if all choral spaces were gender inclusive to the extent that different voice range expectations were separate from the gender of the singers. A treble choir that sings music arranged for sopranos and altos could easily include singers who do not identify as women, with careful consideration for the themes of the repertoire so as not to exclude its nonfemale choir members. Similarly, a women's choir or men's choir could still include all voice parts and perform Soprano/Alto/Tenor/Bass (or Part I/II/III/IV) choral music. Single-gender ensembles can be exclusionary for singers who do not identify within the gender binary, however, and careful consideration for the reasons behind creating a gendered chorus should be given.

CASTING

Casting remains a complex issue when creating gender-inclusive and trans-affirming performance spaces for singers and actors. Although some agencies push for trans inclusion, resistance from studio heads, donors, and producers sometimes prevents progress (Castanho, 2017). Singing teachers who attempt to provide guidance toward a professional career in opera or music theater may find themselves caught between the desire to support their students in their gender journey by training them to play roles that suit their life experience and preparing them for the "real world" where gender stereotypes and typecasting abound.

Casting directors have an opportunity to challenge the gender stereotypes that are traditionally associated with certain roles. There are very few casting calls specifically requesting transgender actors, and in general, audition listings could be worded to be more inclusive of people of all genders. Asking for a "woman in her 20s" or "a male between 35 and 45" automatically eliminates individuals of other gender identities. An improvement on this listing might instead read, "Individuals who identify as gender-masculine, between 35 and 45" or a description of the character with details that may be more relevant than the gender of the actor: "Henry is 35 to 45 years old. He is the strong, silent type who works at the local steel mill. He has trouble expressing his feelings but has a deep devotion to his dog, Jude." The actor receives plenty of information about this character, and if they feel they are able to truthfully convey this person on stage, they should be able to audition for the role regardless of their gender identity.

IMPLICATIONS FOR FUTURE RESEARCH

Repertoire and roles for transgender and nonbinary singers are sparse and difficult to access. Creating a portfolio and building toward a professional singing career can be a unique challenge for trans and nonbinary singers, because the performance industry is still not prepared for gender-diverse talent. Teachers, institutions, directors, and companies have a responsibility to help pave the way for future singers whose identities reside outside the gender binary and whose interpretation of characters and repertoire lies outside the traditional norms.

Future researchers will serve the literature on trans singing by answering questions about how to alter the biases against gender-diverse performers, how to transform traditional works in order to include all gender identities and expressions, and how to create opportunities to amplify trans voices as singers, composers, librettists, directors, and creators. Edited collections of repertoire tailored specifically to the trans experience for several voice types, as well as repertoire designed for nonbinary singers, will also allow teachers to support future generations of gender-diverse students.

REFERENCES

American Idiot LA. (2015, April 20). *American Idiot LA*. Retrieved from https://twitter.com/americanidiotla/status/590278830754 902016

Bornstein, K. (2016). *Gender outlaw: on men, women, and the rest of us*. New York, NY: Penguin Random House.

Broadway.com Staff. (2011, January 18). *Melissa Etheridge to fill in for Billie Joe Armstrong as American Idiot's St. Jimmy*. Retrieved from https://www.broadway.com/buzz/154944/melissa-ether idge-to-fill-in-for-billie-joe-armstrong-as-american-idiots-st-jimmy/

Castanho, C. (2017). Gender diversity in the professional world. *Huffington Post*. Retrieved from https://www.huffingtonpost .com/entry/gender-diversity-in-the-professional-world_us_58 bca155e4b02eac8876d04c

Futterman, E. (2011, February 2). *Melissa Etheridge makes her Broadway debut in 'American Idiot'*. Retrieved from https://www.rollingstone.com/culture/news/melissa-etheridge-makes-her-broadway-debut-in-american-idiot-20110202

Lucas, L. (2017, November 18). Teachers of transgender singers. (L. Jackson Hearns, Interviewer)

Music Theatre International. (2017, December 29). *Pippin*. Retrieved from https://www.mtishows.com/full-cast-info/953

Randel, D. M. (1986). *The new Harvard dictionary of music*. Cambridge, MA: Belknap Press of Harvard University Press.

Stage Agent. (2017a). *American Idiot*. Retrieved from http://stageagent.com/shows/musical/1285/american-idiot

Stage Agent. (2017b). *Pippin*. Retrieved from http://stageagent.com/shows/musical/841/pippin

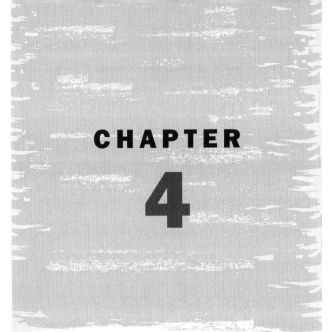

CHAPTER
4

Psychological Perspective:
An Interview With Kelly George
Licensed Clinical Professional
Counselor and Psychotherapist

INTRODUCTION

Because of the personal nature of singing, working with a voice cannot happen in isolation; students must feel seen and understood in order to feel safe enough to make mistakes and grow. Sometimes, it's not a physical or technical limitation preventing students from hitting a high note or successfully executing a musical passage, but a mental barrier, and it takes great bravery and confidence for students to share their learning process and progress with teachers. To develop the full potential of the singing voice, one must be willing to make unfamiliar sounds and learn from their mistakes.

This connection between a person's psychology and their voice plays a large role in voice training. Since there is no exact formula for training voices, the most effective voice teachers take each student's personality, mind-set, and learning style into account when designing their individualized training regimen. So how does this affect the training of transgender singers?

Through the following interview, Kelly George, LCPC, offers insights about the specific needs of transgender and gender nonconforming students. Kelly works in Chicago providing training to businesses, schools, and other organizations on affirmative practices with transgender and gender nonconforming individuals. Kelly's work has taken them to California, Japan, and several places in between. They also teach and provide psychiatric and career counseling at Roosevelt University in Chicago.

Int: indicates the interviewers

KG: indicates Kelly's responses

Int: Can you speak a little about your professional and personal background?

KG: I am a psychotherapist, specifically a licensed clinical professional counselor, at Live Oak in Chicago. I engage in mental health counseling for individuals, couples, and families, and I also do group counseling. I specialize in working with trans and gender nonconforming individuals. I've been running a support group for trans and gender nonconforming folks for about four and a half years now and that has taken on different permutations but is another way in which I support the community. My personal background is that I identify as gender nonconforming and I use they/them/theirs pronouns.

It's been an ongoing and complicated process for myself but I feel that being able to be part of the community that I'm serving, while complicated at times, is also really beneficial. I think it provides me some unique insights into the work that I do. Not that people who identify as cis or straight can't do this work, but just that it's different.

Int: What kinds of mental health challenges do trans and gender nonconforming individuals face?

KG: Trans individuals can struggle with the same mental health things that cis individuals do. Things that anyone can struggle with, a trans person can struggle with. I think there's this perception that people who are trans are somehow sicker, so I just want to acknowledge the reality first. Given the transphobic society that we live in, it's more likely that trans-identified and gender nonconforming folks have gone through some sort of trauma. That trauma could include microaggressions throughout childhood, gender policing throughout childhood, and struggling to maintain relationships with family and friends because of their identity and the reaction of others. These external experiences increase the likelihood of trauma. As trans folks move from these childhood traumas into adolescence and adulthood, you might see experiences with anxiety or depression due to hypervigilance around safety and potential reactionary behavior of other people. Within anxiety as a whole there is a variety of behaviors that can manifest. Anxiety can manifest as a desire to isolate; it can manifest as hyperventilating, racing heart, or panic attacks; and it can manifest as obsessive-compulsive behaviors like counting or hand-washing, to manage the environment and help them feel calmer.

You might also have an increase of depression for some trans folks, especially before they actually self-identify and self-acknowledge that something feels wrong. They may not have a way to describe their feelings beyond sensing that something is off. They might feel sad or angry, but not yet know the real source of those emotions, and their distress comes from not knowing what's wrong, and that's when depression can start to take hold.

Especially during the coming-out process, another source of anxiety can be difficulty in relationships. Specifically, it can be difficult to try to form intimate relationships as a trans person living in a transphobic society. A trans person might come out to someone that they're dating, and even if their social or medical transition process is over for them, the person they're dating might still be reactionary and might not accept them. So that can obviously—or maybe not obviously—lead to feelings of rejection, or dismissal of being able to have intimate relationships.

There's also some discomfort, we call it gender dysphoria, which often relates to the body, but it can relate to other experiences, as well. There is a disconnect; a sense of discomfort and feeling like something isn't right. Some people don't take care of their body very well or are overly focused on their body, some people don't even notice when things happen to their body. They don't know the physical space they're inhabiting because there's such a disconnect. This is especially important for singers, I imagine, when you're asking them to feel their voice or feel something in their body they might react with confusion and skepticism.

Int: How can singing teachers help trans folks feel their body when singing?

KG: Trans folks feel constant and intense focus on their body. People ask about their bodies in an invasive and disrespectful way and there's a sense that they don't have autonomy over their own bodies. For example, in order to get necessary medical services, those who choose to medically transition have to see a mental health professional who then gives permission for them to get treatment. In this way, trans folks aren't able to simply make decisions for themselves and for their own bodies because they want to. The fact that they have to get permission for things like hormone treatments can make them feel powerless about their bodies.

It seems like common practice for voice teachers to need to touch their students and make posture adjustments. When working with trans people, it's important to acknowledge that they may struggle with their bodies and you should be sure to approach touching or decisions about their body in a way that lets them retain and strengthen their autonomy. Always ask if it's OK for you to put your hand on their stomach to show them their breath, or on their head to fix their posture. If it's not OK, ask if you can show them how to do it for themselves. It may feel weird and reductive, but continue to ask until they say that you don't have to ask any more. I have a lot of clients who talk about going to a doctor, for example, who explains everything and asks if it's OK, and they feel so much safer. It feels good to have someone who respects their boundaries and their ability to say "no" without risk of judgment or repercussions. And they may end up being fine with these physical parts of voice teaching, but it's important to let them know what you're going to do, and to be on the same page, showing them that you respect their decisions by asking first.

Int: How can we, as teachers, set up a routine or standard for autonomy for students?

KG: The first step in supporting your trans student and helping them feel their bodies is to set up an environment of safety. Start with a check-in, asking your student about their relationship to their body, what it would be like to do a body scan or if you ask them to feel something in their body. Let them find ways to tell you when that's uncomfortable or too much. Setting up that safety first, letting them know what you're going to be doing, and asking them to let you know when that is—and is not—OK is really important. And if they say that something is not OK with them, stop. Ask if there was something you could have done to make them feel safer, if it's just an off day, or if you took a step too far or missed something.

Once that safe environment is set up, I think with anyone, starting off by asking your student about their connection to their body is a good idea. Asking questions like, "What is body awareness like for you? How aware of and connected are you to your body?" If you're going to talk about using the body and being aware of the body you want to start there. I know breath is very important, for example. I think you could use that, just to have someone practice paying attention, and ask them if they can feel their breath, even just as their sitting or talking. I sometimes do body scans with people and ask if they feel any temperature differences or tension in the body. Just getting them used to feeling their body can be helpful.

Int: Can you talk more about dysphoria? What is it, where does it come from, how does it manifest?

KG: The metaphor that I often give for dysphoria, that a lot of people say they can relate to, is the white noise machine I keep outside my office. When I'm working and making noise I don't hear it but as soon as I'm done it's the loudest thing in the world. And that's kind of what dysphoria is like. Even on days when it's not as bad as others, that feeling of being disconnected is always there. It never goes away, but we create noise or distraction in our lives so that we don't feel it as intensely. A lot of my clients say that the most intense times of dysphoria are when they're alone, when they're going to bed at night, or first thing in the morning. Those are the times when it tends to erupt for them because there's nothing to drown it out. That's why you see people who stay very busy, or use drugs or alcohol or different ways to try to self-medicate that disconnection.

Being trans doesn't inherently mean that you hate your body. It may mean that you have a complex relationship with your body. It may mean that some days your body feels really comfortable and safe, and some days your body feels like a betrayal—that it's not doing what it's supposed to do. I think for trans people that are more binary-identified, there is more of a sense that their body is not the way that it should be, or the way that would be the most comfortable for them to move through the world. For people that are more gender nonconforming, it can be more mixed. Some days they may feel really great about their body and then maybe small inter-actions will happen and they feel suddenly very uncomfort-able. I had one client who was talking about how they're generally pretty disconnected from their body in a lot of ways, and they were at an event and someone grazed their chest, and they immediately became completely overwhelmed and shut down. It made them aware of a part of their body that they're uncomfortable with. So especially if you're thinking that you're going to be touching someone on the torso, that tends to be an uncomfortable area for a lot of people. It may be a part of their body from which they're completely discon-nected, and then suddenly you're asking them to connect to it and they may say, "I don't know if I can do that."

Dysphoria means different things to different people, and it's definitely something you could check in with. The loud-ness or prevalence of it varies based on experiences and things going on throughout the day. Asking your students what role dysphoria might play in lessons, asking them to communicate when they're having a more dysphoric day so you know to touch them a little less or maybe you're a little less focused on their body that day, is a good way to support them.

Int: Is there such a thing as vocal dysphoria?

KG: Yes. I would define it as a sense that someone's voice does not match how they want to present themselves in the world, or that the way they hear their voice in their head doesn't align with what is coming out, or maybe that they don't have a problem with their voice, but the way other people hear their voice leads people to constantly misgender them or treat them differently.

Int: Is that part of why a trans person might resist taking up space with their voice or being heard?

KG: Especially people that are binary and want to pass, they may want to be invisible. They don't want to be seen—they want to just blend in and pass, and if they're not passing yet, they want to blend in as something else until they can flip a switch and be seen the way they want. That's not how transition works, unfortunately. I can't tell you how many clients say, "If I could just go away to an island for 2 years and come back and be this new person, that would be amazing," because everyone is terrified of the in-between. The most anxiety-provoking, difficult time is the time between "I've decided to medically transition" and "I feel like I pass." For some people that time period is a couple of months, for some people that period is 2 years, and it's scary because that's a time when they're most likely to have violence enacted against them. I think especially if you're working with someone who is in the midst of that process, understand that for them it's scary to be visible and to have their voice be heard. They feel very vulnerable and exposed already, and now you're possibly asking them to expose themselves even more and that can be terrifying.

Int: Is it important for someone's voice to align with their identity?

KG: It's very important. I think it's the individualized, personal nature of it. For some people, the priority is in getting a voice that helps them pass and helps them feel safe in the world. For others, it's about finding a voice that is authentic, regardless of whether they pass. I think it's a matter of pulling those things apart for people. They may want to have a voice style for when they're with their friends and/or for when they're in a situation where they're surrounded by strangers and want to move through the world without anyone questioning. Someone might say they want a voice that is authentic and feels really good, and also that they want a voice that keeps them safe, and those might not be the same thing for everyone. Especially thinking about someone living in an area that's much less accepting than Chicago, they may need that voice so they can go into a job interview and secure employment. Having a voice that "matches" can mean different things to different people and it's important to recognize that and be open to it.

Int: We've had fellow teachers ask us about repertoire and roles for their performance majors. We want to encourage and support these students, but how do we start having this dialogue about casting, auditions, and repertoire?

KG: There might have to be some reality testing and managing expectations. You might have to tell your students that with their voice in this way, they may not be able to do certain parts. And that, I imagine, you have to do in general. Somebody says they want to sing alto and you have a conversation with them about what their voice can do. Talk with them about what their voice range is, their capacities and limitations, and what parts they can have. Explore that together, brainstorm together on finding pieces that work for them, or how to manipulate pieces so they work for your student. Where are places that your trans singer would be more accepted and where are places that they wouldn't? If you're working with stage singers, for example, the difficult part will be figuring out what role they will play on stage, what they are comfortable doing, and how they are going to present themselves based on where they are in their transition. So, let's say you have someone that was assigned female at birth and is starting to present as more male but most people still interpret that person as female. How are they going to go into an audition? How will they present themselves? Taking time to have that discussion and ask your student what that will be like for them will help you make decisions together about songs, roles, auditions, etc. Some people will say they want to take time off until they pass, and that has to be OK, too.

You can actually use these kinds of conversations to further affirm your student. I think about cabaret singers and how often they'll work with a musician to change the key so that they can sing the repertoire. I'm using terms I don't really know, but they might take a song that was written for a man and put it in a different key, or shift lyrics around so they can sing it. Talk about the history of that with your student, let them know that this isn't just trans folks; singers in general have done this for ages and ages. Another thing that I have found helpful for my clients is tapping into music that brings them closer to their ideal sound. For example, they could listen to female singers that have a deep voice and embrace it, singers who make that their signature. A lot of jazz singers have a deep, smoky, "masculine" voice but they were known for that and it was a powerful thing for them. Help your student to find examples of nontrans folks and trans folks as best you can that fit their voice style. Reassure them that they're not the only one who sings this way; lots of people sing this way. Ask them what it would be like for them to hear somebody else singing like that.

Int: What are some obstacles to getting voice training?

KG: I think honestly the first obstacle is financial. Medical transition is expensive and can include accessing hormones, cosmetic services, surgery, name change, clothes, all of that. In addition to cost, trans folks may not have access to employment during their transition because, again, we live in a transphobic society. They're having to pay for hormone therapy, pay for doctor's visits, pay for mental health care possibly, and those costs add up. For a lot of my clients, their first reaction is that they can't afford voice lessons.

Once they can feasibly budget for voice lessons, then I think there is a concern about whether the person they're going to see is trans-affirming. They might be asking themselves, "Is this voice coach or teacher going to remove my autonomy and tell *me* what it means to be a man or a woman?" It's important for vocal coaches and teachers to be open to asking students what they want their voice sound like, what their ideal might be, and making a plan to help them achieve that, rather than strictly prescribing a "male" or "female" voice. And the students may not know, and you can coach them a little bit from there, figuring out what they do or don't like, what sounds good to them. Saying, "OK well I'll just teach you how to be a woman" is the wrong attitude. It's one of the most frustrating things for the trans folks that I work with and they tell me, "I'm tired of people telling me how to do this, and telling me this is the right way to do this. You're doing it wrong." They are looking for someone to have that flexibility, knowing that they can go somewhere and someone will ask them, "What's your voice? How do we find that?"

Int: What are some important things to have in mind when deciding to take on a trans client?

KG: I think two things. I think be honest with yourself about whether you can actually do the work to be good to trans folks. And if you can't, be honest about it. If it turns out you're just not willing to do it, that's on you and not the trans person. The second piece is the self-reflection piece—are you willing to do this work? Are you willing to change, or at least reevaluate, your own ideas about gender and voice to create an environment where your trans clients can flourish?

My partner is in a choir and they're starting to move away from men's choirs and women's choirs and instead go by part, like here are the altos and here are the sopranos. She has found that that's more helpful anyway, because you can't know what someone's voice is based on their gender. Even for somebody that's cis, you may think that woman probably sings really high and they actually sing really low. So moving away from saying "singing with the girls" or "singing with the men" and talking more about "singing with the altos" and actually using the terminology, moving away from gendered language, is a great way to be more inclusive.

The other thing to keep in mind is that pronouns are so important and you have to get it right. And when you get it wrong, you have to acknowledge it and talk about it. And if you mess it up a lot, you need to really go within yourself and decide what are you doing wrong. Trans folks are not always going to correct you because it's exhausting, and sometimes there's a concern that it will get overblown by the person who made the mistake. If someone uses the wrong pronouns with me, and they say, "I used the wrong pronouns I'm sorry, I really meant they," that's just fine. But if it's, "Oh my god I'm *so sorry!* It's just so hard I'm sorry," on and on, now I have to hold their shame and fix it and tell them that it's OK. It's not OK, but I have to tell them it is so they'll shut up about it. Rather than making a big deal of it, it's better just to acknowledge it and then move on. What I prefer is if someone says, "Oh Kelly she did—I mean they did this the other day" and fix it immediately and then keep going.

If you keep messing it up, you may need to have a conversation with your student, and it's not an excuse to say that it's really hard for you. You know what's hard? Being trans. That conversation needs to sound more like, "I'm sorry, I'm really working on this. Can we talk about how you could correct me, or how we can make a space where I can correct myself?" Have an open conversation about it if you're struggling with it. But keep in mind, if you're struggling with it, there's something going on. You're still connecting your expectations in your head of gender to your language and to that person. You have not yet separated the gender expectations from what you see. You have to pull apart visual perception and identity, and probably also what you hear and how that manifests as gender expectations.

Int: What would you say in response to folks who might resist asking all their students for their preferred name and pronouns when they sign up for lessons?

KG: I would present it as, "I'm starting to work with folks whose pronouns are not always immediately apparent to me. You may think that it should be immediately apparent to me what your pronouns are, but I'm asking everyone to be respectful because I don't want to make any exceptions." At Live Oak, we ask all of our clients what their pronouns are, and I had to push really hard for that. And now, it is no big deal and we haven't lost any clients for it. I also like to ask people about their preferred name because some people like to go by a nickname or their middle name. I just want to make sure that I'm referring to my clients in a way that feels comfortable for them. And cis people will sometimes still even say, "I hate being called ma'am" or "I hate being called miss" or "don't call me honey." You're just being respectful of all the ways someone wants to be addressed, even beyond pronouns.

Int: Gender-neutral pronouns seem to be a sticky spot for some people. Can you talk a little about the importance of singular *they* as a gender pronoun for an individual and about your own choice to use singular *they*?

KG: Gender-neutral pronouns, and specifically singular *they*, have been in existence in our language for a very long time. Chaucer and Byron, who we think of as the paragons of language, used singular *they*. So that's not out of the ordinary. Similarly, there was panic about moving away from using *thou* and using *you* instead, but now it's commonplace. The other interesting thing is that people use singular *they* a lot; they just don't realize it. For example, if a friend and I walked into a room and we saw somebody's cell phone, I might say, "Oh no someone left their phone here, I wonder if they know that they left it. Do you think they'll call it?" And we wouldn't even think about it, because we don't know the gender of the person so we just automatically use singular they.

Singular gender-neutral pronouns allow space for those of us who do not identify as part of the binary. In my own personal experience, although I was assigned female at birth I have never identified entirely as being female or with what was expected of me with that role. All throughout my life, even early childhood, there was a disconnect between the expectations of me being a girl my experience of my own gender. When we would play house, I wouldn't be the mom or the dad or the child. I would be the dog. My mom likes to tell the story that even when I was an infant I would cry and kick whenever she would try to put me in a dress. I did the same thing for shoes, of course, but I like to tell the story with the dresses. And she thought it was funny too, until I came out as gay.

I have always presented as masculine; I was a tomboy as a kid and I just never grew out of it. In college, there came a point when I realized that clearly my masculinity is important to me and something I want to embrace. I started redefining myself and my gender expression by cutting off my hair, wearing men's clothes, things like that. When I came to Chicago, I started doing drag performance and I was a drag king for several years. At that point, I started to ponder whether I actually identify as a man. I was going through a lot of internal processing, thinking about moving through the world being seen as a man, but in the end, that didn't feel comfortable for me either. So truly, for me, I identify strongly as both woman and man. I feel, and have felt, an intense connection with women and that's important to me, but I also feel a very deep connection to my own personal sense of masculinity. And what that manifests as for me is an internal sense of strength and other various aspects of my nature.

My partner actually instigated my switch to *they/them* pronouns. When we started dating, one of the first questions she asked me was "What pronouns do you use?" and I said, "Uh . . . actually I've been thinking about *they/them*, but you could use *she/her*." And then she said, "Well, I'll use *they/them*." She was the first person to use it consistently with me and that felt really good and really affirming. And then I asked a few more friends if they would try it out, and eventually I realized that when people used *they/them* I felt seen and understood. I had felt all my life that my masculinity was bad, that it was something I was supposed to hide, that it wasn't OK for me to have, let alone OK for me to embrace. I was only positively reinforced when I was acting feminine and embracing that. When people use *they/them* pronouns with me it's like there's finally breathing room, that I can embrace both masculine and feminine and that's OK. And people see that, and they see me as more than just one or the other because I am more than just one or the other. Gender-neutral pronouns are important to me because they help me to move through the world as a whole person and let other people acknowledge that wholeness and unity versus forcing me to divide myself. It's important to other nonbinary people because they want to be seen and understood, and they want to know that there's a place for them in the world and *they/them* pronouns help begin to carve out that space. Pronouns aren't the only thing, but they're a big thing.

Int: The decision for trans masculine folks to take testosterone, or T, is a pretty weighty one. How can we help and provide appropriate guidance through that medical transition?

KG: The level of education that you provide to your students, knowing things about hormones and voice that your student's other health providers don't, is great. When I started learning more about voice and transition, being able to tell my clients what I learned was really helpful. It was great to be able to tell my clients that the reason why so many trans men end up with a scratchy voice is because their vocal cords are getting thicker and bigger, but the space that they're in isn't. All the education that you can put clients through about the biology of their voice, and what will happen, and what the plan will be, is empowering. Giving them really concrete plans and expectations, when all the aspects of transition are not concrete, can make a big difference in that decision to go ahead with T or not. They may not know how long some things are going to take or what's going to happen, but this is pretty clear-cut.

In addition to being super educated, you can help them do preparatory work before they start testosterone in order to have a more natural voice during and after medical transition. From what I've learned, doing some of that preparatory work can deepen their voice quicker and keep it more flexible. Liz and I shared a client who is a singer and started T over a year ago, and I noticed he had a quicker change than I would have expected. I wondered how much of that was him embracing it as it was happening, and if people that aren't doing that aren't having that same rate of change or comfort or malleability. There was a period of time, and this might or might not happen to everyone, but he was losing the top end and not gaining the bottom end yet so his range was just shrinking and that was scary for him. Voice lessons helped him through it and that was so empowering to him. To know that things would change, that it was stuck temporarily, but that those low notes were going to come helped him feel a lot calmer about it. When his range started expanding he was like, "Oh thank god. My teacher was right!" From that one experience, I saw how vocal coaches that have a firm understanding of the biology of what's going to change and what's going to happen to the voice and to the body in ways that will impact the voice is really important. Because there's so little concrete knowledge from which to draw comfort, when you can give just a fragment of that it's so meaningful. We're so hungry for knowing what happens to our bodies when we start hormones, and being able to assuage that at all is powerful.

Int: So many people are doing this voice work by themselves. How do we reach out the folks who feel alone?

KG: For so long, knowing where to get resources, knowing how to embrace your identity, knowing how to transition, was all held in the community. As a trans person, we would find someone who could give us information about which doctor to go to, or find the one person who's figured out how to pass and they would teach other folks how to do makeup. The information has been kept within the community, and we've been teaching each other how to do things. The problem is that without access to experts, we're just doing it as best we can and then passing along that information. Especially with the advantage of the Internet, the first thing people do is go online and google "trans voice" and they look at forums, YouTube videos, and blogs, and people talk about what they've tried that has worked or hasn't. There are so many YouTube videos of people talking about how they pitch their voice and pass, but they don't know anything about voice health and they don't know anything about how to sustain that kind of voice. They're trying to be helpful, but people in the community don't know that there's anything else. There's a sense that the only people who will help are the other people in the community.

Part of creating a positive, trans-affirming environment is about giving away information and building trust in that way. And then from there, individual people will seek you out as an expert because obviously you know what you're talking about and you get how to be trans-affirming. As an expert, if you can connect with someone in the community and show them that you are trans-affirming, they'll pass on information about you to other folks. Eventually, by word of mouth, you'll start to develop that network and the community will be reassured that you get it and they'll start to come to you for voice. Most people just go online first to figure out the voice work until they learn they have other options, but without the guidance from experts, it could be—and ultimately often is—more damaging.

Int: How do teachers get to the trans communities and find more trans students?

KG: My first recommendation is to volunteer and give out free information as much as possible, to build trust and build relationships with individuals. Find your local LGBTQ organization and offer to do free voice workshops and give out free information in exchange for leaving your marketing materials there or getting listed on their website. I think also reaching out to professionals who are working in the community is a good idea. I have a good professional relationship with a couple of voice teachers here, so we have frequent opportunities to cross-refer. Reach out to mental health professionals who specialize in gender identity. Reach out to doctors who specialize in medical transition; they are hungry for these resources so let them know that you're available to provide information about voice. Also connect with lifestyle providers like hair and makeup artists, electrolysis places, and gyms.

Int: How can we learn more about trans experiences while we build up those networks? Where is the boundary between presumptuous and invasive versus helpful?

KG: When you live in a city there are panels, for example, Center on Halsted does panels all the time with trans folks, and that's a totally appropriate time to learn about trans people. You could also look for trans movies, books, articles, YouTubers, etc. to learn about trans identity that way. Even if you're not talking directly with trans folks, look for places where they have invited the audience to learn more about them. I think if you have a close friend, you could ask for permission to talk with them about their transition, but keep in mind they may say no. Most people would probably be OK, but some might say that they don't want to talk about it. If you frame your questions in such a way that lets them know you're trying to have a better understanding of this experience, they'll probably be more open with you. Be compassionate about it, and rather than questioning their identity or asking questions like, "How did you know" instead say, "Tell me what this is like for you." I think people tend to feel a little attacked sometimes when they get asked questions like, "How did you know you were trans?" Those types of questions can sometimes come from people who are questioning themselves, and then they pry into other trans people's lives and don't know how to handle it. And that's not fair to anyone.

There are always more things to learn. I don't know it all, and I've been doing this work for years now. I identify as part of the community, and I learn something new every day. This is a constantly evolving field because only within the last 10 to 15 years has there been any degree of visibility, and we've seen a drastic increase within the last few years. In creating a trans-affirming space for your students, be open to learning, being wrong, making mistakes, and be open to people telling you you're making a mistake. Rethink your language. I'm constantly having to rethink my language to find the best ways to say things. I will screw it up, and when someone lets me know that I've made a mistake I thank them and try to adapt and change and be better. But if your response is resistance and stubbornness, then you'll lose people, and that's sometimes irreparable. I want to reiterate that you have to really evaluate whether you want to do this work. If rethinking your language and being open to adaptability isn't something you think you can do, then don't do this work.

Int: What resources do you recommend for learning more about trans identity?

KG: When people ask me about resources I usually go on Amazon and look at the newest stuff that has good reviews. There are a few staples that I really like, though. There's a compendium book that I think is really wonderful called *Trans Bodies, Trans Selves* [Laura Erickson-Schroth, 2014]. Although it's a good resource, there isn't a lot of information about voice. Some people may be more interested in the medical component and should look up journal articles. From there I think personal stories are really good. Janet Mock's book *Redefining Realness* [Mock,2014] is great; I also really like *Meet Polkadot* [Broadhead, 2013] and *Gender Outlaw* [Bornstein, 2016] and other books like that. I think Kate Bornstein's really wonderful; I also really like the author of *Stone Butch Blues*, Leslie Feinberg [Feinberg, 1993]. They wrote a book called *Trans Warriors* [Feinberg, 1996] about what's happened to trans communities over time. For young folks, watching a video of someone talking about their experiences is very meaningful and helpful. Just meeting trans people and talking to them and getting to know them and hear about their experiences is a good way to learn. You don't want to use people as a zoo, of course, but talking to folks about their own experiences can be helpful.

Int: What else do you want us to know?

KG: I want to make sure that the readers know that yes, being trans is hard. There is difficulty and there are scary things that happen. And it's also beautiful and there is rewarding, empowering work you can do. I think especially being a voice teacher, allowing someone to have their voice is amazing. To give voice to someone who may have felt silent for a long time, whether it's because they didn't know how to express themselves or because they were scared to use their voice because it didn't match, is special. To let someone open up and express themselves, that's just amazing. I get to do that in the sense of giving them their voice and giving them language to talk about their experiences. It's just as important to give them the kind of voice you do, too.

So many of my clients are musicians and music is a way for them to process these experiences and talk about what's happened to them and talk about their gender and what that means to them. Thinking about the client Liz and I shared again, we were able to complement each other because I would challenge him to write songs about what he was thinking about what he was going through as a way of processing. What does it mean to become a man and what does that mean to him? And that was one of his favorite songs, the one he wrote about that process. So many of my clients use music and singing to bring forth that emotion and break out of that silence and bring forth who they are and manifest that. It gives them so much confidence. The work you do is so needed and they will be so appreciative of it in ways that I don't think you'll experience with anyone else. If you can do this work, it'll be some of the most rewarding work you'll ever do.

RESOURCES

Bornstein, K. (2016). *Gender outlaw: On men, women, and the rest of us.* New York, NY: Penguin Random House.

Broadhead, T. (2013). *Meet Polkadot.* Olympia, WA: DangerDot.

Bunch, M. A. (1997). *Psychological aspects of singing.* Vienna, Austria: Springer.

Erickson-Schroth, L. (2014). *Trans bodies, trans selves a resource for the transgender community.* New York, NY: Oxford University Press.

Feinberg, L. (1993, 2003). *Stonebutch blues.* New York, NY: Alyson Books.

Feinberg, L. (1996). *Transgender warriors: Making history from Joan of Arc to Dennis Rodman.* Boston. MA: Beacon Press.

Mock, J. (2014). *Redefining realness: My path to womanhood, identity, love, and so much more.* New York, NY: Atria Paperback.

Taylor, D. C. (1908). *The psychology of singing.* New York, NY: Macmillan.

PART TWO

The Voice

Respiration and Special Considerations for Transgender Singers

My housemates don't know that I am trans. . . . I walk around the house with my chest poked just that little bit further out. I hold my head up high, but low enough to hide my Adam's apple. As much as I pride myself on gender [screwing] and confusing people, I am constrained by my need to protect myself.

—Nyah Harwood, *Trans Bodies, Trans Selves* (p. 137)

INTRODUCTION

Connecting the voice to the body is one of the foundational principles of voice pedagogy. Breath is the "motor" of the voice, and efficient vocal production is difficult if not impossible to achieve without adequate and appropriate breath technique. Singers constantly seek out new ways to free the body through movement, mindfulness, imagination, exercise, body mapping, gesticulation, or any of a number of other methods (Neely, 2012). Respiration is a fervent topic of discussion among voice teachers, and despite differences in opinion or approach, teachers usually agree that breath technique is important.

Trans and nonbinary singers face unique challenges in the realms of body awareness and respiration. Dysphoria can be a source of discomfort, leading to dissociation from the body, or hypervigilance, which makes connecting to the body difficult or anxiety inducing (Reynolds & Goldstein, 2014). When working with trans and nonbinary singers, reframe questions or instructions for respiration and body connection to encourage autonomy and agency on the part of the singer. This chapter outlines specific challenges trans singers face when developing breathing techniques and suggestions for maneuvering those challenges to help singers find more comfort and release.

BODY-SHAPING GARMENTS

Transgender and gender nonbinary individuals sometimes wear body-shaping garments to change their appearance and find relief from symptoms of dysphoria, including the sense of incongruence about one's body as an expression of gender identity (Reynolds & Goldstein, 2014). Chest binders diminish the appearance of breasts, and waist trainers create an hourglass curve through the torso and waist. Both types of garments have been used in performance settings for centuries, usually worn for several hours and then removed or taken off. For transgender and gender nonconforming individuals, however, a chest binder or corset becomes part of the daily wardrobe (Peitzmeier, Gardner, Weinard, Corbet, & Acevedo, 2017). It may seem difficult to imagine wearing a constricting garment every day, but it is important to keep in mind that for many people, physical discomfort is preferable to extreme mental and emotional discomfort.

Singing with constrictive garments around the rib cage and abdomen may present challenges for respiration, intonation and pitch control, registration, dynamics, or overall vocal function by limiting movement of the ribs, diaphragm, and abdominal muscles. Chronic tension in the back, shoulders, or neck may interfere with the singer's ability to find ease in voice production or could even prevent concentration and attention. Changes in blood flow to different parts of the body, including the brain, compromise the singer's stamina in musical phrases and length of practice or lesson time (Gau, 1998). Figure 5–1 depicts some of the impact a body-shaping garment could have on movement of the ribs and diaphragm.

Despite the challenges mentioned above, going a day without a binder or waist trainer has equally dangerous consequences. Trans people may fear being misgendered because of the contour of their body in everyday scenarios like grocery shopping, using the restroom or locker room, or even walking down the street. Being "clocked" as trans, or not passing can result in social rejection, ridicule, or physical violence. In addition to perception of gender by the outside world, inward psychological and emotional distress from dysphoria and the sense of incongruence about one's body can cause a great deal of discomfort (Reynolds & Goldstein, 2014).

Singing teachers have an opportunity to support students through aspects of transition, including decisions about garments like chest binders and waist trainers. To show a student that they can sing and discover freedom in musical expression while still presenting in ways that give them confidence and security is deeply meaningful. For the reasons listed above, it is not appropriate to ask a student to remove their chest binder or waist trainer at any time, nor is it appropriate to criticize or punish them for the decision to wear body-shaping clothing. Teachers should navigate the differences that body-shaping garments present, helping students find vocal freedom alongside their gender expression.

Talking With Students About Constrictive Garments

Students may share their experiences about wearing a chest binder or waist trainer, or they may prefer not to discuss it. The decision to wear body-shaping garments, as with all other aspects of social and medical transition, is deeply personal and it is important to respect each student's decisions and follow their lead in discussion. Directly addressing

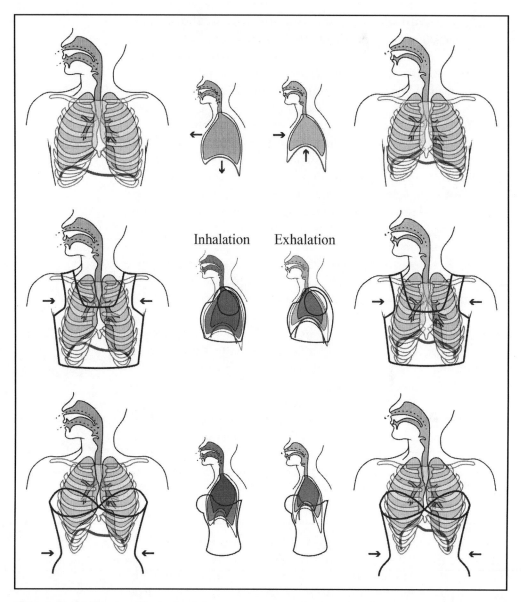

Inhalation   Exhalation

Figure 5–1. Effects of body-shaping garments on respiration. *Top:* No body-shaping garments. *Middle:* Chest binder. *Bottom:* Corset.

body-shaping garments in an accusatory or insensitive way could compromise trust. Additionally, people who experience gender dysphoria about their bodies may be hesitant or uncomfortable with exploring sensations of breath. When asking students to connect with their body, it is best to show respect by asking permission first rather than giving direct instructions.

> ## Box 5–1. Questions to Ask Your Students About Body-Shaping Garments
>
> "What would it be like to feel your breath in your body?"
>
> "How does your breath feel today?"
>
> "Do you notice any tension or restriction anywhere in your breath?"
>
> "What is it like to release your abdomen and allow the breath to be free?"
>
> "Would it be OK if I put my hand on your back/ribs/shoulders/etc.?"
>
> "What would it be like to place your hand on your own stomach/ribs/chest to feel your breath?"

Chest Binders

The appearance of breasts can immediately influence the gender perception of an individual. For trans men, trans masculine or nonbinary people, chest binders prevent others from immediately identifying them as female or feminine. Binders, sometimes called compression tanks, fit tightly around the chest; some extend from the shoulders to just below the rib cage, and some extend the full length of the torso. Binders are made from stretchy compression fabric or layered mesh, similar to a sports bra but typically more constrictive (Peitzmeier, Gardner, Weinard, Corbet, & Acevedo, 2017). Prior to the common use of chest binders, many folks who wanted to change the appearance of their chest used sports bandages or tape to bind their breasts, but it is not advisable to use these methods. Binding in this way can significantly irritate the skin and prevent any mobility in the rib cage, which can be dangerous (Reynolds & Goldstein, 2014). Unlike a chest binder, which returns to its shape with movements of the body, a sports bandage constricts even tighter after it has been stretched. In an extreme case, using a sports bandage could crush the singer's rib cage or damage internal organs. If a student binds their chest using tape or bandages, discuss options with them and see if using a chest binder instead is possible.

Chest binders are available for purchase through several different stores, and there are multiple resources and discussion forums led by trans masculine individuals who provide reviews and personal experiences about different types and brands of binders. Table 5–1 includes a short list of binder types and retailers.

Because chest binders are tight and restrictive, long-term wear can produce some negative side effects for the wearer. Some people report breast tissue bruising, rib cage bruising or soreness, stomach pain when wearing a full-torso compression binder, pain in the shoulders and neck, misalignment of the spine or other back pain, and dizziness or difficulty breathing (Peitzmeier et al., 2017). Some health professionals and other trans men suggest binding only 8 hours per day; even this amount, worn every day over the course of months or years, can add health risks and side effects for the individual (Wesp, 2017). It is important to remember that despite these side effects, reshaping the contour of the chest is worth the discomfort for many individuals.

Binding for Singers

Chest binding is not a new practice in the world of singing; many singers who have breasts have used binders to portray a masculine or gender-neutral character and give the appearance of a masculine physique on stage. In such instances,

Table 5–1. Types of Binders and Retailers			
Retailer	**Binder Type**	**Colors**	**Cost (USD)**
GC2B	Half binder	Black, white, gray, red, blue, olive green, various shades of nude	$33
GC2B	Full binder	Black, white, gray, olive green, various shades of nude	$35
f2mbinders.com (Underworks)	Compression postsurgical vest	White	$28–$35
f2mbinders.com (Underworks)	Compression tee shirt	White, black	$31–$38
f2mbinders.com (Underworks)	Compression tank	White, tan, black	$18–$38
Shapeshifters	Chest binder tank	Various colorful patterns	$45–$50
Venus Envy	Cotton-lined chest binder	White, black	$50

singers wear the binder only as long as is necessary for the production, perhaps only for a few hours at a time. For a trans masculine singer, however, the binder is not a temporary accessory but a necessary undergarment.

The restrictive nature of a binder can prevent diaphragm and/or rib movement and thereby prevent a full, expansive breath. In turn, the singer may have trouble with various aspects of singing, including pitch control, sustaining long notes or phrases, or difficulty maneuvering registers. Some trans masculine singers wearing binders report a lack of dynamic control or general lack of vocal "power." If a singer is unable to manage breath efficiently, they may become dizzy or light-headed and need to take frequent breaks. Tension in the back, shoulders, and neck sometimes occurs, and this tension can translate readily to laryngeal or extralaryngeal tension as well, which can limit vocal flexibility and stamina. A singer's posture may also become difficult to maintain, which can exacerbate these tension issues.

Box 5–2. Carl

After several months of testosterone, Carl's high range was still easily accessible because he had been using his voice regularly. During one lesson, he was focused on successfully singing through a particular musical passage that required some amount of dynamic control. He sang through the phrase a few times, but he started looking a little pale. He said he was dizzy, so he sat down and let the dizziness pass. His hydration, nutrition, and general vocal health were all normal, but it seemed that he had overexerted himself.

He said he was having trouble taking in a deep breath and he knew his chest binder was preventing his ability to breathe well. After discussing a few options for what to do through the rest of the lesson—he could continue singing while sitting down, take a break for a few more minutes, or work on a different part of the song for a while—Carl asked if he could go to the restroom and loosen his binder. None of the options presented for how to continue were related to binding, but he elected to loosen the binder of his own accord. He came back a few minutes later with color in his cheeks again and returned to singing, now with a little more ease and flexibility.

> ## Box 5–3. Liam
>
> *In developing a deeper resonance, Liam had been learning to open his throat and body more and imagine his sound vibrating through his chest. In one lesson, it was obvious there was some stiffness during breathing. It had not come up in conversation yet, but it seemed clear the stiffness was because he was wearing a chest binder. He said that his abdomen felt tight and he utilized some body mapping exercises to help loosen the tension and allow for a lower breath. After asking about whether some of his clothing might be restricting his breath, he mentioned the chest binder and that although he doesn't wear it as tight as some people do, it was likely still restricting. He decided to focus on maintaining looseness in his abdomen so that he could still breathe relatively easily, despite the restriction on his rib cage from the binder.*

Top Surgery

Some trans and nonbinary individuals eventually opt for mastectomy, commonly called "top surgery." Top surgery can be an expensive procedure, as with many other aspects of medical transition, but has a high success rate and the individual's feeling of relief postsurgery is significant as well (Peitzmeier et al., 2017).

> ## Box 5–4. Ashton
>
> *Ashton sought out voice lessons before he started testosterone and was able to move through his medical transition with a team of professionals supporting him. In his first lesson, he said that he had been binding for several months already and was noticing some health problems. More than once, he came to a lesson having recently seen a medical professional about some of the side effects of binding that were affecting his shoulders and spine. He talked about it openly and was enthusiastic about finding solutions to make his breathing life easier, but still things were tough. Eight months after starting testosterone therapy, Ashton had trouble with dynamic control,*

long phrases, and maneuvering through registers. Part of that difficulty was the progression of voice change through hormonal transition, but he knew part of it was his binder. He eventually elected to have top surgery and recovered remarkably quickly. His confidence and happiness went through the roof, and he was back in lessons 2 weeks after surgery. The difference was incredible. Not only did he have better breath management and dynamic control, but he found new ways to access his high register and gained flexibility and control seemingly overnight. A few months after surgery, he recorded his first full-length album with a healthy voice.

Box 5–5. The Singing Teacher's Perspective

Liz: As voice teachers, we hear our students' voices as though we were experiencing them ourselves, and this enables us to help them make decisions about technique. I found myself at a loss when working with my trans masculine singers because I had never sung with a binder before and didn't have that mutual feeling to draw from and give guidance about. I decided to acquire a chest binder and experience singing while wearing one.

After buying from a recommended retailer, spending 10 to 15 minutes putting it on for the first time, and adjusting to the redistribution of fat and skin in my torso, I was ready to sing. Immediately after putting the binder on, I could feel that my breath was limited. My ribs could barely move and even so it was like pushing against a barrel of tightly bound wood. The binder only extended to just below my rib cage, which left my abdomen somewhat free to move, but my abdomen also felt distended from being tightly bound just above it. My posture was abnormal as well; there was more skin under my arms than normal and my shoulders were hoisted from underneath. Simultaneously, the tank straps pulled down in front and it was difficult to maintain an open chest.

Warm-ups and vocalises were manageable, to an extent, but the points along my range that require the most breath and dynamic control—the passaggi—were nearly impossible to manage. I approached the passaggi as I knew how to and my voice cracked, wobbled, deflated, went out of tune, or just stopped altogether. I had limited access to the lowest parts of my range, which I cherish, and it was at first quite distressing. Even singing into the most upper parts of my range, which were easier, quickly exhausted me. Though the singing was challenging, gaining insights from using a chest binder has been invaluable. Continued use and support from Brian led me to discover ways to compensate for my compromised body and breath system, though it became clear that singers who use chest binders regularly likely spend a great deal of concentration on maintaining the most basic vocal functions.

Waist Trainers

Waist trainers and corsets have seen a resurgence in popularity recently by female celebrities, inspiring women to adopt this potentially dangerous body-altering technique. Waist training is a process by which the corset wearer increases the tightness of the corset to the desired, smaller, waist size. The result is a temporary change in outward body shape but could be a permanent change in bone structure, muscle strength of the back and abdomen, and alignment of internal organs (Fee, Brown, Lazarus, & Theerman, 2002). For singers, corsets can displace the diaphragm and misshape the rib cage, significantly decreasing lung capacity and breath control (Gau, 1998). Waist training may also increase digestive problems, which could exacerbate vocally disadvantageous conditions such as acid reflux (Gau, 1998). Even with these risks in mind, however, trans and nonbinary people sometimes choose this body-shaping technique in search of relief from dysphoria.

Types of Waist Trainers

Corsets and waist training methods are available from a variety of sources and in a variety of styles. Commonly, waist training corsets are made from stretchy, breathable fabric with hook-and-eye closures and extend from the hips up to the bra line, and different kinds of boning like plastic or metal allow for different levels of flexibility in the corset. Some methods of waist training recommend using a nonbreathable material such as plastic wrap to improve efficacy of the technique, but use of these materials can be damaging to the skin and come with other side effects (Peitzmeier et al., 2017). Table 5–2 includes various types of waist trainers/corsets and retailers.

Corsets for Singers

Like chest binding, singers have performed in corsets for centuries (Neely, 2012). Corsets affect respiration by limiting movement of the diaphragm and lower rib cage and by limiting the displacement of internal organs during inhalation and exhalation (Gau, 1998). Singers wearing corsets may need to concentrate movement of respiration toward the upper ribs, accompanied by relaxation of the shoulders, back, and neck. This method of upper-body breathing may affect the singer's ability to find the stability necessary to sustain long phrases, extend vocal range, or achieve balanced phonation. When discussing options for breath management with singers, it is not appropriate to ask them to remove their waist trainer, but talking with them about navigating some of the challenges of body-shaping garments gives students the opportunity to make the best decision for themselves.

Table 5–2. Waist Trainers/Corsets and Retailers

Retailer	Corset Type	Material	Colors	Cost (USD)
Lucy Corsetry	Round Rib	Cotton, steel boning	Various	~$100
Lucy Corsetry	Conical Rib	Cotton, steel boning	Various	~$100
Lucy Corsetry	Cincher	Various	Various	$75–$80
Angel Curves	Extreme Waist Trainer 2 and 3	Latex exterior, cotton interior	White, black, "nude," animal print, lace	$59–$65
Angel Curves	Gym Waist Trainer	Lycra/Latex, flexible boning	Pink, blue, red, black	$59
Angel Curves	Waist Training Vest	Latex exterior, cotton interior, flexible boning	"Nude," black	$74
Angel Curves	Zip-And-Clip Non-Latex Waist Trainer	Lycra, cotton	Black, lace	$65

> ### Box 5–6. Lorraine
>
> *Lorraine was an active person who loved sports in addition to singing. She had trouble sometimes being still long enough to focus on breath but made significant improvement after years of lessons. She usually wore a spandex corset and high heels to lessons, both of which sometimes prevented her from finding restful poise and easy breathing. She could only sing short phrases and had limited control through passaggi and in head voice, although her goals included developing her upper registers to sound bright and shimmering.*
>
> *After talking through some of the mechanics of breathing and learning how the corset might be interfering, she decided to utilize the spandex around her waist as a way to improve control and strength through her abdomen. Simultaneously, she learned to release some tension in her shoulders and back in order for her rib cage to move more freely. She practiced slow, rhythmic breathing and started to gain more conscious control of her rate, volume, and frequency of breaths. Along with that progress came more control through her middle range and freedom in her upper notes, though she remained an active and fluid singer, humorously unable to stand or sit still for very long.*

Body Alignment and Respiration Without Body-Shaping Garments

Some singers who do not choose to wear body-shaping garments may still show signs of manipulation of their physical appearance through postural habits. Trans men or trans masculine people may not be immediately comfortable fully expanding into their breath for fear of showing a feminine contour in their chest. Trans women or trans feminine singers, influenced by societal pressure to maintain the appearance of a flat stomach and petite figure, may be reticent to allow relaxation in their shoulders or abdomen because it may feel as though they are demonstrating a masculine-perceived body type. Conversely, many transgender individuals have felt pressure to outwardly demonstrate the gender they were assigned at birth in order to fit in, and creating new habits of body alignment may feel unnatural or inauthentic. Using questions like those listed in Box 5–1 that begin with "what would it be like to . . . " rather than simply instructing the student to explore realigning their body can mean the difference between comfortable breathing and anxious, restricted breath.

FINDING SUCCESS THROUGH THE CHALLENGES

Although chest binding and waist training can cause stress and challenges for a singer, there are ways to maneuver through these demands to ensure the health, well-being, and vocal success of the singing student. Discuss the side effects and difficulties of singing while wearing body-shaping clothing with the student with patience and compassion.

In some breathing methods, singers attempt to expand the rib cage as much as possible, and some teachers encourage the use of resistance training (wrapping a scarf or belt around the rib cage, attempting to hold the ribs out as long as possible) in order to build stamina. For the singer using a chest binder or waist trainer, this is not advised. Emphasis on pushing the rib cage out may cause rib, abdominal, and/or chest tissue bruising and do much more harm than good. Instead, encourage the student to maintain tensile looseness so that the abdominal muscles can release and allow some diaphragm movement, and the ribs can move more freely.

Limited movement of the breath mechanism can also make long sung phrases difficult. Allow the singer to add musical breaths or pauses when needed, and segment long phrases into smaller, more accessible parts. Respiration exercises in Appendix 3 encourage the singer to maintain flexibility and buoyancy in the breath while also building necessary stamina for long, held notes.

Keep aware during lessons if the singer becomes dizzy or light-headed and allow time for breaks. If the student complains of physical pain or discomfort while singing, evaluate the source of the discomfort and discuss options. Some body-shaping garments are adjustable with hook-and-eye closures or Velcro; it may be beneficial to loosen the garment while singing, especially if the student experiences these side effects regularly. Discuss options with the student and allow them to make their own best decisions regarding body-shaping garments.

REFERENCES

Deutsch, M. B. (2017, January 1). *Binding, packing, and tucking*. Retrieved from http://transhealth.ucsf.edu/trans?page=guidelines-binding

Fee, E., Brown, T. M., Lazarus, J., & Theerman, P. (2002). The effects of the corset. *American Journal of Public Health, 92*(7), 1085.

Harwood, N. (2014). The shower. In L. Erickson-Schroth (Ed.), *Trans bodies, trans selves: A resource for the transgender community* (p. 137). New York, NY: Oxford University Press.

Peitzmeier, S., Gardner, I., Weinard, J., Corbet, A., & Acevedo, K. (2017). Health impact of chest binding among transgender adults: A community-engaged, cross-sectional study. *Culture, Health, and Sexuality, 19*(1), 64–75.

Reynolds, H. M., & Goldstein, Z. G. (2014). Social transition. In L. Erickson-Schroth (Ed.), *Trans bodies, trans selves: A resource for the transgender community* (pp. 124–154). New York, NY: Oxford University Press.

Wesp, L. (2017). *Transgender patients and the physical examination*. Retrieved from http://transhealth.ucsf.edu/trans?page=guidelines-physical-examination

CHAPTER

6

Hormone Therapy and Voice

My mental changes have come drastically in such a short time. I already feel much more confident, and much more in tune with my body, like a missing piece has finally been put back in its place.

—Patient quote, *Trans Bodies, Trans Selves* (Deutsch, 2014, p. 251)

INTRODUCTION

Before even uttering a sound, assumptions about a person based on their physical appearance allow the brain to automatically and subconsciously categorize input, specifically related to gender. For a transgender or gender nonconforming person, aligning physical appearance with gender identity makes it easier to move through the world authentically by aligning that person's hormone levels and affecting their body appearance to be more congruent with their identity. Development of hair or breasts, changes in distribution of muscles and fat throughout the body and face, and voice changes all occur when someone undergoes hormone therapy (Deutsch, 2014). These changes in body shape, facial appearance, voice, and mood can bolster the confidence of someone experiencing dysphoria and improve quality of life (Unger, 2016).

Not all trans people choose hormone therapy, but those who do understand the significance of the decision as it relates to voice. Unfortunately, trans people are not always supported by a unified health and voice care team to help them make the best decisions for themselves. Included in this chapter is information about the various hormone therapies available to trans individuals and their effects on the body and the voice. This information can help equip the singer for important conversations with their endocrinologists and other health professionals about hormone therapy.

MASCULINIZING HORMONE THERAPY

Trans men experience gender policing beginning early in life, especially if their social circles encourage stereotypically feminine socialization for folks who are assigned female at birth. Regardless of presentation through clothing, hairstyle, mannerisms, speech patterns and word choice, or social behavior, it can take the final addition of testosterone to alter their appearance and the sound of their voice enough to be seen and heard fully as themselves. The decision to initiate testosterone therapy can only be made by the student and their physician, but providing knowledge to the student about how testosterone might affect their voice supports those discussions with health care professionals and arms them with agency through education.

Many trans masculine singers have reservations about beginning testosterone therapy because of the potentially limiting and irreversible effects on the voice. Others may be eager to begin hormone therapy in order to find alignment between their gender identity, expression, and perception. There are several types of masculinizing hormone therapy regimens. With guidance and prescription from a trusted health care provider, individuals may begin masculinization hormone therapy as early as adolescence (Unger, 2016).

Several types of testosterone delivery are available:

- Injectable testosterone, either intramuscular or subcutaneous
- Testosterone patch
- Testosterone gel
- Oral testosterone

Source: Transgender Health Information Program British Columbia (Provincial Health Services Authority, 2017).

Effects of Masculinizing Hormones on the Body

As early as 6 to 8 weeks after beginning testosterone therapy and continuing for up to 2 years, several physical changes take place. Facial hair begins to grow, the jawline changes and becomes more defined, fat begins to dissolve under the skin and relocate throughout the body giving a leaner appearance, menstruation ceases, the skin and hair become oilier, and male pattern baldness begins to appear (Deutsch, 2014; World Professional Association for Transgender Health, 2017). Many of these changes, including voice changes, are irreversible even after stopping testosterone (Adler, Hirsch, & Mordaunt, 2012).

Testosterone therapy affects the individual's entire body and can have negative side effects, including water retention, fatigue, mood swings, and general aches and pains (Deutsch, 2014). Testosterone can also affect kidney and liver health, affect cholesterol, or increase the risk of certain types of cancer. Providers may perform regular tests for liver and kidney health, diabetes, and ovary and uterine health during therapy (Unger, 2016).

Effects of Masculinizing Hormones on the Voice

The physiological changes to vocal fold tissue during hormonal transition are significant. It is reasonable, but inadequate, to compare a trans masculine person's hormonal journey to that of an adolescent whose body naturally produces testosterone. During adolescence, increasing levels of testosterone change the mass and length of the vocal folds, and the cartilages of the larynx grow larger, resulting in a lower pitch range and deeper resonance (Titze, 2000). For those who receive testosterone from an outside source, this process occurs in part. The vocal folds increase in mass and the pitch range of the speaking and singing voice drops, which is the desired result for many people engaging in testosterone therapy (Davies & Goldberg, 2006).

Some trans masculine individuals are concerned with how much and how quickly they will observe changes in their voice during hormone therapy. For singers, however, prolonging the voice changes can help maintain vocal health and elasticity as the vocal folds increase in size (Constansis, 2008). Constansis (2008) states, "Abrupt changes are rarely beneficial to the vocal instrument. Even in a flexible adolescent laryngeal structure with gradual hormonal changes, the voice is rendered uncontrollable and of limited use for a certain period of time." (para. 9). The same holds true, perhaps even more so, for trans males. Constansis advocates for gradual progression of testosterone when possible, to support transition into the singer's new range and give time for adjustments in resonance and registration management while the physiology of the vocal folds and larynx changes.

Singers whose bodies produce testosterone naturally experience the same gradual shift in vocal range, accompanied by simultaneous shifts in laryngeal cartilage structure. The difficulty for trans and nonbinary singers who undergo testosterone therapy after adolescence lies in the incongruence of vocal fold mass and laryngeal cartilage size. Because many trans masculine people begin hormone treatment after adolescence, the laryngeal cartilages cannot grow large enough to adequately accommodate the vocal folds (Constansis, 2008; Davies & Goldberg, 2006). Testosterone therapy is also known to cause early ossification of the cartilages in the larynx, and the ossification process happens abruptly because the onset of hormonal change is more sudden than for people whose bodies produce testosterone naturally (Adler et al., 2012). A stiffer, less pliable laryngeal structure can limit vocal fold movement significantly, preventing control of dynamics and difficulty navigating a new pitch range. Constansis (2008) calls this phenomenon "entrapped vocalization," and the resulting tone is characterized by hoarseness, weakness, or rough voice.

Refer the student to a laryngologist and/or speech pathologist if roughness in the voice persists.

Another change to prepare for during hormonal transition is adjustment and descent of the larynx within the throat, although the degree or extent of this change can vary widely between individuals (Adler et al., 2012). For some singers, a lower larynx position could be disorienting as they attempt to maintain healthy techniques appropriate to the genre. For others, a lower larynx position provides the opportunity to create a deeper, more masculine-perceived voice quality with a longer vocal tract and deeper resonance. Maintain open conversation about how these adjustments arise in the student's voice, and give room for the student to express discomfort or concern while working through this realm of vocal transition.

Amid these abrupt and irreversible changes to vocal fold physiology, testosterone therapy may provide some vocal health benefits. Addition of testosterone to vocal fold tissue increases the production of hyaluronic acid and fibronectin, which heal and rebuild the vocal folds (Mukudai, et al., 2015). "Male" (testosterone-laden) vocal folds contain more hyaluronic acid than "female" (estrogen-laden) vocal folds, which helps maintain optimal thickness of the outer layer of the vocal folds (Titze & Abbott, 2012). In short, testosterone therapy may help to make the vocal folds more resilient during or after voice change.

Ultimately, the singer and their health care provider will make the best choice for the individual; singing teachers can offer information about the effects of testosterone hormone therapy on voice, but it is inappropriate to make outright medical recommendations for the student. And regardless of the ease with which testosterone is introduced, there will still likely be a period of vocal instability, for which teacher and student should prepare (Davies & Goldberg, 2006; Irwing, Childs, & Hancock, 2017).

Box 6–1. Eli

Eli began voice training approximately 8 months after starting testosterone. He received injections every other week—to be more accurate, he injected himself every other week. When he started lessons, he shared that his friends and colleagues often asked if he was ill because his voice was hoarse and husky, though easy to perceive as a masculine voice.

He had very little control of his singing voice and often had difficulty with pitch-matching. Tuning was a challenge for him since he had never sung in this new pitch range and was still navigating his new voice after starting medical transition. He also had a unique quality to his voice and some difficulty maneuvering registers. There were several notes in the middle of his range that he could sing with either a light, falsetto-like quality or a heavier, thicker quality, but not with anything in between. Sometimes this either heavy-or-light production shows up in his voice still, but less often. In other circumstances, a messa di voce exercise might help bridge the gap between these two types of sounds, but unfortunately Eli had neither the control of his pitch nor his breath yet to work in this way.

Considering that a trans masculine person's vocal folds change physiologically in such a way that they can become very stiff and unmalleable, he decided to work on creating a healthy sound before maneuvering dynamics or register management. He spent quite a bit of time using straw phonation and other semi-occluded techniques and over time some of the coarseness of his voice started to dissipate. At one lesson, he walked into the room and proclaimed proudly that no one asked if he was sick at a party he had been to the night before. It took several months of voice work, but eventually he found a more reliable voice production. In those months, he stayed with the same dosage of testosterone and his voice began to settle and smooth out.

Box 6–2. Ray

Ray began androgen therapy treatment 13 years prior to his first voice lesson. At his first meeting, he complained about his singing and speaking voice lacking in power. When he began to sing, he had a vocal range of only about five to six notes, and the head voice/falsetto was completely inaccessible and produced only as air. When asked about this, Ray explained that before hormone therapy, he had a lovely head voice and soprano range, but he had severe dysphoria attached to its sound. He described it as "foreign" and like "something that didn't sound like me." He wanted to rid himself of it as quickly as possible and find a timbre that he felt best expressed his gender identity.

He began to find this voice during hormonal transition. He described "pressing" his voice lower as his vocal folds were changing to try and access the lower parts of his voice faster. He enjoyed his new range and felt more like himself. However, during the transition, he paid no attention to his head voice and had no assistance from a voice teacher or another voice professional to aid in making this change as healthy and smooth as possible. Most likely, the combination of "pressing" the voice, ignoring the head voice, and lacking professional supervision is what caused his lack of vocal power and range.

After 3 months of lessons, Ray's voice grew in size and range only moderately. In his haste to deepen his range, he may have created an irreversible hurdle to his vocal training that he will continue to work through for years.

Singing Through Masculinizing Hormonal Transition

During hormonal transition, most singers experience a period of time when the voice is unpredictable and shrinks in singable range. According to Constansis's own documented experience, this holds true even when the singer adheres to a strict vocal practice and voice health regimen (Constansis, 2008). Frequent changes to aspects of voice, including range and voice quality during hormonal transition, can be expected, at least for the first 12 months (Irwing et al., 2017). During this time, the singer will likely experience some stress and worry about the health of their vocal instrument, but knowing what to expect can often assuage some of those anxieties. Figure 6–1 delineates voice ranges over time during hormonal transition for six different transgender male or nonbinary singers, ages 21 to 44, at varying stages of testosterone treatment.

Changes in pitch and voice quality begin as early as 6 weeks after the start of hormone therapy, even on a gradual dosage plan, and may not plateau or finalize for 2 years or more (Irwing et al., 2017). During this time, the singer's voice range may descend anywhere from a few semitones to an

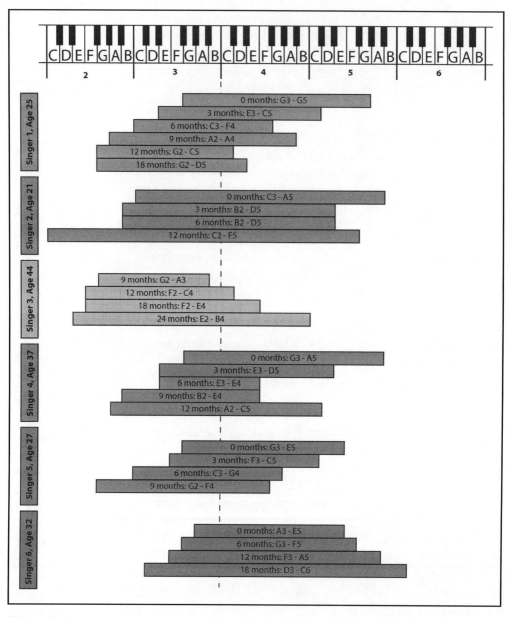

Figure 6–1. Rate and extent of voice change during testosterone hormone therapy. All but Singer 3 began voice training prior to engaging in testosterone therapy.

octave or more (Adler et al., 2012). Maintaining exceptional vocal health and continuing to use upper registers during vocal exercises will help maintain elasticity in the vocal fold tissue and may help prevent hoarseness or total loss of upper register notes (Constansis, 2008). During such exercises, continue talking with the student about vocal dysphoria; regardless of the vocal health benefits of maintaining an accessible upper range, it may be too psychologically uncomfortable to approach those areas of voice without first discussing it and gaining permission from the student. Revisit that discussion often while exploring different realms of voice range extension.

The most difficult period of hormonal transition seems to be approximately 4 to 6 months after beginning testosterone treatment. At this point, the singer's voice is at its weakest and may have a very narrow range. Sadly, this is a time when some singers abandon lessons and resign to permanently losing their singing voices. Reassure the student that this is an anticipated phase in the vocal journey and that they will regain those minimized parts of their range, at least to some degree. During this time, it could be useful to work through nonphonatory aspects of singing such a breath, articulation, interpretation, and developing good mental practice habits.

Once the voice has settled during the period of 8 to 24 months after starting treatment, positive improvements to voice range and voice quality can be expected. Some singers not only observe lower pitches in their habitual speaking range and singing range but are able to retain relatively high pitches as well, increasing the usable singing range significantly (Constansis, 2008).

In addition to working within a new pitch range, singers in hormonal transition may also struggle with maneuvering registers and passaggi. Lower or heavier register voice production involves thick vibration of the vocal folds (Titze, 2000). Because the transitioning singer's vocal folds have greater mass than before, this production is sometimes the easiest, although often still accompanied by hoarseness due to vocal fold swelling. Lighter productions require the vocal folds to vibrate on a thin edge (Titze, 2000). These types of vibration patterns are much more difficult for transitioning singers to achieve once vocal fold changes have begun. Sometimes the heavier and lighter voice productions are irrevocably separated and divided by a large gap in the passaggio near middle C (Constansis, 2008). Exercises that would benefit any other singer with this difficulty would also benefit a singer in hormonal transition, with the knowledge that the relationship of vocal fold size to larynx size may be somewhat incongruent or limiting for those types of exercises.

Transitioning singers also sometimes have trouble creating high-amplitude vibration in the vocal folds. To create loud sounds, the vocal folds vibrate with increased amplitude of oscillation, aided by increased lung pressure (Titze, 2000). For some, achieving this increase in amplitude is difficult because the larger vocal folds simply have no room left before reaching the maximum possible oscillation amplitude. To visualize this scenario, imagine a pair of hands inside a small shoebox; it would be difficult to clap loudly because the movement of the hands would be limited by the walls of the shoebox. This issue is often compounded by the use of a chest binder, preventing maximally efficient breath management for singing. The ability to sing comfortably loudly and to have control of vocal dynamics is vitally important for proficient singing and can be challenging after the student has begun hormone therapy. *Messa di voce* and other exercises that explore changes in dynamics may be helpful to encourage flexibility and stamina in breath management and dynamic range.

Despite the potential setbacks and side effects, many trans masculine singers are enthusiastic about beginning hormone therapy and about the changes they will see and feel in their body and voice. Supporting a singer through this process can be an enlightening and challenging experience for both teacher and student, provided that both understand and seek out research and education about the changes to come.

Box 6–3. Ashton

Ashton began his voice training shortly before starting testosterone treatment, though he had already decided that testosterone therapy was the right choice for him. With excitement, he discussed some options and how he might start his medical transition and what his goals would be. He wanted a lower voice and a more masculine appearance, both of which he knew would be accessible with testosterone. Ashton kept his voice team informed of the decisions he and his medical providers made and about any changes in dosages or side effects.

He noticed one of the first side effects after beginning "T" was water retention. Ashton's legs and feet were swollen, and he started showing signs of vocal fold swelling: delayed onset phonation, squeakiness, and difficulty maneuvering into his upper registers. After the first month, Ashton noticed his voice beginning to change more dramatically. His total singing range lowered and he gained a few semitones at the lowest part of his range. His voice continued in this way for another month with very little trouble, while keeping much of his upper range as well.

During the period of 4 to 6 months after the start of hormone therapy, a significant portion of his singing range disappeared. His speaking voice was unsteady and cracked often. His singable range decreased to the narrow interval of a sixth, and rather than gaining any notes in either direction in his range, it seemed he was losing more notes all the time. He tried reparative voice techniques like straw phonation, but his vocal folds were too swollen to handle the increase in phonation threshold pressure. Other semi-occluded vocal tract exercises, including humming and using fricative consonants, made some improvement. He spent a great deal of time practicing vocalises, which Ashton was patient to continue with even through his anxiety. Still, he was discouraged. He continued to talk openly about his stress and used Constansis's data as a reference for tracking his own vocal journey. It was a rough time for him, and it is a time during which many singers give up.

By the time Ashton had been on testosterone for 8 months, his voice began to settle. His speaking voice was still gruff, but it cracked less often. He recovered notes above middle C and gained several more in his low range. Between 8 and 12 months after starting hormone therapy, he gained more flexibility between registers and could reliably move through all the parts of his range, which was still growing. Ashton had top surgery 10 months after starting testosterone, which helped him gain more control and stamina.

Now, a few years after the start of his hormonal transition, Ashton's voice is steady and he continues to gain strength and control in his upper and middle ranges. The richness of his voice is improving and he's discovering new ways to play and balance resonance to find his own unique, free sound.

FEMINIZING HORMONE THERAPY

The pressure to exhibit traditionally feminine characteristics can be a heavy burden, especially for singers. In auditions, at performances, even in rehearsals there are sometimes expectations for dress code, makeup, and general presentation that permeate a female singer's daily life. Trans women feel that pressure to a magnified degree because for some, their bodies have naturally produced testosterone for years, leaving them with physical features that are not congruent with a feminine-perceived presentation. That incongruence is painful and distressing. Hormone therapy can provide relief of the distress of dysphoria by realigning some of the physical characteristics that are influenced by the presence of different hormones in the body.

There are a few basic combinations of feminizing hormone therapies, listed below (Provincial Health Services Authority, 2017). Common regimens include:

- Estrogen only (Estrace or Estradiol)
- Estrogen with testosterone blockers (Estradiol with Spironolactone or Finasteride)
- Estrogen with testosterone blockers and progesterone (Estradiol, Spironolactone, Medroxyprogesterone)
- Testosterone blockers only

Source: Transgender Health Information Program British Columbia.

Effects of Feminizing Hormones on the Body

Each individual experiences the physical changes that accompany feminizing hormone therapy differently. Commonly, differences in skin tone are among the first noticeable changes; the body produces less oil, skin may be more prone to bruises or cuts, and the odor of sweat or urine may change (Deutsch, 2014). Within a few months, additional modifications begin to emerge. The skin softens; fat redistributes into the hips, thighs, and buttocks; breasts develop; muscle mass decreases; facial and body hair decreases; and some people feel a change in emotional state as well (Deutsch, 2014; World Professional Association for Transgender Health, 2017). These changes begin within the first 6 months of beginning feminizing hormone treatment and continue for up to 2 years. Many of the physical changes return to their previous state if hormone treatment stops (Provincial Health Services Authority, 2017).

Negative side effects of feminizing hormone therapy may include weight gain, edema, migraines, mood swings, or hot flashes. Increased blood pressure, cholesterol, and risk of blood clots may also accompany hormone treatment. Health care providers maintain and track information about hormone levels, kidney and liver function, and screen for diabetes during therapy (Unger, 2016).

Effects of Feminizing Hormones on the Voice

Changes in hormone levels affect the entire body, including vocal fold tissue. Increases in estrogen and decreases in progesterone can cause vocal fold swelling and production of thick, viscous mucus (Kadakia, Carlson, & Sataloff, 2013). This may affect the ability of the vocal folds to vibrate freely with sufficient lubrication and could lead to decreased stamina and risk of cell damage to the outer layer of the vocal folds. Administration of estrogen hormone decreases the presence of fibroblasts, the cells responsible for repairing and rebuilding tissue in the vocal folds (Mukudai, et al., 2015). This could mean that trans women are more prone to vocal fold damage after beginning hormone replacement therapy.

In adult trans women whose bodies produced testosterone during puberty, increases in larynx size and shape and vocal fold size and length have already occurred and are irreversible (Davies & Goldberg, 2006). The addition of feminizing hormones has not been shown to significantly alter the physical structure of the larynx, voice range, or color of the voice, though it could be inferred that reduction in the muscular content of the vocal folds would positively affect the singer's ability to create a lighter sound, if desired (Schneider & Courey, 2016).

Despite the lack of significant change in vocal range or timbre, the psychological and emotional shifts that occur as the student's appearance aligns better with their affirmed gender can be helpful. Increased confidence can certainly play an important role in improving voice health and ability to take on new techniques.

Box 6–4. Allie

Transition is a difficult experience, especially for vocalists. Allie began hormone therapy only a few weeks before seeking out voice training. Her vocal identity was fraught with stress and confusion as she weighed her options. She began working on resonance and inflection to expand her vocal color palette as she considered what a more feminine singing voice meant for her.

Allie's mood when she began voice work was low and there were periods of despondency. Her voice was one small piece of the many difficult aspects of transition and of redefining her outward identity to express who she felt she was. Estrogen hormone therapy seemed like the first step, but there were so many more. Each week she trudged into her voice lesson, apologizing that she hadn't practiced much but promising she would do better. It was clear that continuing voice lessons was as much about Allie creating a safe and supportive space for herself as much as it was about voice education. She talked about some of her vocal idols, discussed how femininity might show up in her voice and what that meant, and worked to develop confidence that she had full control of her voice goals and had no one to please but herself. It wasn't immediate, but over time she began to claim her transition and truly blossom.

She remained on estrogen for the next several months and noticed her features beginning to change and soften. She began carrying herself differently. Her improved posture helped with breath management as well as ease throughout her upper range. Where before there was rigidity and hopelessness, confidence and flexibility emerged. She was finally able to explore and play with her voice—not because her voice changed, but because the hormone therapy started to change her appearance and her self-confidence skyrocketed. Over time, she made some decisions about her voice and chose to stay in a gender-neutral range. Having the freedom and support to make her own choices, supported by the desired effects of her hormone therapy, she was confident enough to use her voice in the ways that she wanted.

RECOMMENDED READING

Chyten-Brennan, J. (2014). Surgical transition. In L. Erickson-Schroth (Ed.), *Trans bodies, trans selves: A resource for the transgender community* (pp. 265–291). New York, NY: Oxford University Press.

Gorin-Lazard, A., Baumstarck, K., Maquigneau, A., Gebleux, S., Penochet, J., Pringuey, D., . . . Bonierbale, M. (2012, February). Is hormonal therapy associated with better quality of life for trans-sexuals? A cross-sectional study. *Journal of Sexual Medicine, 9*(2), 531–541.

Irwing, M. S., Hancock, A., & Childs, K. (2016). *Testosterone therapy and the female-to-male transgender voice: A prospective study* (pp. FRI-134). Boston, MA: Endocrine Society.

White, H. J., & Reisner, S. (2016, January). A systematic review of effects of hormone therapy on psychological functioning and quality of life in transgender individuals. *Transgender Health, 1*(1), 21–31.

REFERENCES

Adler, R., Hirsch, S., & Mordaunt, M. (2012). *Voice and communication therapy for the transgender/transsexual client: A comprehensive clinical guide* (2nd ed.). San Diego, CA: Plural.

Constansis, A. N. (2008). The changing female-to-male (FTM) voice. *Radical Musicology, 3*, 32 pars.

Davies, S., & Goldberg, J. (2006). *Trans care: Changing speech*. Vancouver, Canada: Trans Care Project.

Deutsch, M. (2014). Medical transition. In L. Erickson-Schroth (Ed.), *Trans bodies, trans selves* (pp. 241–264). New York, NY: Oxford University Press.

Irwing, M., Childs, K., & Hancock, A. (2017, January). Effects of testosterone on the transgender male voice. *Andrology, 5*(1), 107–112.

Kadakia, S., Carlson, D., & Sataloff, R. (2013, May/June). The effect of hormones on the voice. *Journal of Singing, 69*(5), 571–574.

Mukudai, S., Matsuda, K. I., Nishio, T., Sugiyama, Y., Bando, H., Hirota, R., . . . Kawata, M. (2015, March). Differential responses to steroid hormones in fibroblasts from the vocal fold, trachea, and esophagus. *Endocrinology, 156*(3), 1000–1009.

Provincial Health Services Authority. (2017, January 1). *Transgender Health Information Program*. Retrieved from http://transhealth .phsa.ca/medical-options/hormones

Schneider, S., & Courey, M. (2016, June 17). Transgender voice and communication—vocal health and considerations. In M. Deutsch (Ed.), *Guidelines for the primary and gender-affirming care of transgender and gender nonbinary people* (2nd ed., pp. 161–171). San Francisco, CA: Center of Excellence for Transgender Health.

Titze, I. R. (2000). *Principles of voice production*. Iowa City, IA: National Center for Voice and Speech.

Titze, I., & Abbott, K. V. (2012). *Vocology: The science and practice of voice habilitation*. Salt Lake City, UT: National Center for Voice and Speech.

Unger, C. A. (2016, December). Hormone therapy for transgender patients. *Translational Andrology and Urology, 5*(6), 877–884.

World Professional Association for Transgender Health (WPATH). (2017, January 1). *Standards of care for the health of transsexual, transgender, and gender nonconforming people Version 7.* Retrieved from https://s3.amazonaws.com/amo_hub_content/ Association140/files/Standards%20of%20Care%20V7%20-%20 2011%20WPATH%20(2)(1).pdf

Pitch and Registration

When you're a trans woman, you are made to walk this very fine line, where if you act feminine you are accused of being a parody, but if you act masculine, it is seen as a sign of your true male identity. And if you act sweet and demure, you're accused of reinforcing patriarchal ideals of female passivity, but if you stand up for your own rights and make your voice heard, then you are dismissed as wielding male privilege and entitlement.

—Julia Serano, *Excluded: Making Feminist and Queer Movements More Inclusive* (pp. 28–29)

INTRODUCTION

Regardless of genre or singing style, the goal of a singer is to achieve a vocal quality and artistry that is both natural and authentic. For the trans singer, however, the meaning of those two terms may be in flux or may require reevaluation. How does one define a "natural" sounding voice or an "authentic" voice? Are these two qualities interdependent? A singing teacher might define a natural voice as one that sounds free and unfettered by tension or apprehension that expresses both mastery and musicality. An authentic voice reflects and upholds a composer's intentions through accurate and thoughtful interpretation. A trans singer might add that a natural voice sounds personal and reveals genuine emotion but that an "authentic" voice sounds like it was born to sing in the chosen style, voice range, and voice quality. It is not a consistent or absolute opinion, but some trans people feel pressure to find a voice that sounds as though they were born as their affirmed gender and that only then will their voice be authentic. The pressure to "pass," even in singing, is prevalent and can be challenging.

Fear of being perceived as fake or as a caricature of one's gender can influence decisions around gender expression and presentation. Altering gender presentation to be more congruent with one's identity, or *transitioning*, is a complex and personal process, and often voice is a significant part of transition (Reynolds, 2014). If a trans person decides to incorporate voice into transition, they are actively defining their own natural voice, with the goal of developing an authentic presentation of their gender. If a singer chooses to change or experiment with their singing voice, the goal is the same: to discover a voice that feels as though it truly belongs to them and that it expresses who they are. This chapter includes information about pitch range and registration unique to trans singers and encourages teachers to manage students' expectations while also supporting them as they define vocal success for themselves.

PITCH

Vocal attributes such as pitch range, registration, resonance, and articulation give cues, or *gender markers*, about the perceived masculinity or femininity of a voice. A trans student has likely been studying such gender markers already, but they may not know which gender markers appear in their own voice or which aspects of perceived gender they might want to shift in their singing, if any. Perhaps they would like to maintain the same pitch range but develop darker resonance or learn how to extend their upper range and sing a higher voice part, or perhaps the singer's interest is in claiming and enjoying their entire voice range in fluid and exploratory ways. It is important to strike a balance between the student's voice range goals and the potential limitations of the instrument. Follow the student's lead about which parts of their voice they are comfortable investigating and developing, but ensure vocal health and sustainability of techniques.

Pitch is among the most prominent and salient gender markers in voice that listeners hear and categorize automatically and subconsciously. Low-pitched voices are generally perceived as more masculine and high-pitched voices more feminine (Adler, Hirsch, & Mordaunt, 2012). Voice range holds great significance to singers while developing artistic identity, but gender-conscious voice training dispels any associations between pitch range and gender. A high- or low-pitched voice range does not determine, and is not necessarily related to, the singer's gender identity.

Some transgender people feel most comfortable and confident in specific parts of their voice range, even throughout the process of dissociating voice range from gender expression. Because pitch is a concrete, definable, and easily measurable aspect of voice, it can be a source of immediate feedback for some singers, for better or worse. Singers may compare their current voice range to others and place unnecessary pressure on themselves to conform or align with the voice range that "matches" their gender. This may not always be the case, however, and for those students, unlocking vocal production over their entire range feels just as organic.

Table 7–1 shows voice ranges for 20 transgender singers alongside their voice parts in an all-transgender chorus. It is interesting to observe the distribution of gender identities across all voice parts in this choral atmosphere. In Chapter 3, Table 3–1 illustrated sample voice ranges and genders for different voice parts. Such tables are typically used to guide teachers toward repertoire choices and pedagogical objectives, using pitch range and gender as criteria for determining next steps for the student. Table 7–1 illustrates that these guidelines are less useful in a gender-inclusive studio environment; the gender of the singer may have nothing to do with voice part.

Table 7–1. Pitch Ranges and Voice Parts of Singers in an All-Transgender Chorus

Singer	Pitch Range	Voice Part	Gender
Singer 1. Age 28	A2–F5	I (high)	Male
Singer 2. Age 32	C3–C5	I (high)	Male
Singer 3. Age 29	C3–C5	I (high)	Nonbinary
Singer 4. Age 25	F3–F5	I (high)	Nonbinary
Singer 5. Age 40	C3–F5	I (high)	Female
Singer 6. Age 40	D3–F5	I (high)	Nonbinary
Singer 7. Age 38	G2–G4	II (medium high)	Nonbinary
Singer 8. Age 21	C3–F4	II (medium high)	Nonbinary
Singer 9. Age 20	E3–C5	II (medium high)	Nonbinary
Singer 10. Age 42	A2–G5	II (medium high)	Female
Singer 11. Age 45	G2–C5	III (medium low)	Male
Singer 12. Age 65	G2–D4	III (medium low)	Male
Singer 13. Age 19	B3–G5	III (medium low)	Male
Singer 14. Age 35	C3–C6	III (medium low)	Nonbinary
Singer 15. Age 29	A2–A4	IV (low)	Male
Singer 16. Age 46	F2–D4	IV (low)	Male
Singer 17. Age 39	G2–B4	IV (low)	Female
Singer 18. Age 60	F2–A4	IV (low)	Female
Singer 19. Age 34	B2–E4	IV (low)	Nonbinary
Singer 20. Age 55	G2–A4	IV (low)	Female

Singers should have opportunities to make unique and personal choices about the ways in which they use their voices. For example, a trans woman may learn to speak in a pitch range that is perceived as feminine during her transition and still choose to sing low-voice repertoire. Her speaking voice keeps her safe and lets her express herself as she moves through the world in daily life, but as a singer she has the artistic flexibility to retain her low singing voice if that feels natural and healthy for her. As discussed in Chapter 6, estrogen hormone therapy has little known effect on the voice range of a trans singer. The decision to sing in a high or low voice range in this singer's case relies on the capabilities of her instrument, her own strengths and dedication as a singer, and her skilled and supportive teacher. Discussing the student's artistic identity and their relationship with their voice is a constant process to be undertaken without judgment and with persistent encouragement toward freedom.

Box 7–1. Jenny

One of the wonderful things about an all-transgender choir is the flexibility to deconstruct traditional voice parts and any accompanying gender associations. Before beginning her medical transition, Jenny had a lovely, rich bass-baritone voice. During her time in an all-trans choir, Jenny has freely explored many different voice parts and eventually decided to stay in the low range, although she has a great deal of strength in her upper range. Jenny's speaking voice is smooth and feminine, and she is quite fond of the richness in her voice. Singing remains a joyful activity and she has autonomy and freedom to sing the parts in choir that she enjoys and performs well.

Box 7–2. Flora

Flora began her voice training as a nonsinger hoping to gain more confidence in her speaking voice. Because she had experimented with voice work on her own before starting lessons, she already knew that pitch is only one part among the series of gender markers within voice and communication. Flora also enjoyed karaoke and decided she might like to sing more formally and joined an all-transgender choir. Presenting as female in her voice, whether singing or speaking, was a high priority for Flora. Even as she acquired skills beyond pitch change to influence gender perception of her voice, she remained focused on increasing her upper singing range. Choosing songs that kept her from singing in the lower parts of her range was important because it was a source of dysphoria and discomfort. For her, singing low pitches was foreign and inorganic—it wasn't her voice. The reactions she had when exploring notes below middle C might have been similar to any other soprano in the same range. Her facial expressions changed and she was visibly uncomfortable and described the lower part of her voice as "weird and heavy."

Despite the challenges, and supported by her own decision making about songs and repertoire, Flora stayed dedicated to singing. As her singing voice began to unlock and open, she was able to navigate through some of the tongue and jaw tension that had made its way into her speaking voice. The skills she learned to aid her in healthy singing also supported her speaking voice, and she started feeling more confident. Even now, her goals still include increasing her pitch range and letting go of tension as she aligns her singing voice more with her speaking voice (or perhaps vice versa). Pitch range extension is an important aspect of her singing journey that she continues to expand, with reasonable expectations and a great deal of patience with her own instrument.

Each singer must be given autonomy over decisions about which voice ranges to explore, without assumptions surrounding pitch range or voice part. It should not be assumed that a singer who identifies as male or masculine is interested in singing in a low pitch range or that a feminine or female singer is interested in a high pitch range. To discover and invest in a natural, authentic voice requires constant reevaluation of goals and priorities for the student and teacher.

Box 7–3. Eli

Singing was not a passion of Eli's before he began medical transition, and he did not go through hormone therapy with the same concerns or preparation as a career singer might. Eli began singing as a hobby, several months after he started testosterone therapy, and his voice was quite low already. Pitch was the most important part of voice training for Eli when he first started singing. At each lesson, he was excited about reaching low notes and was reluctant to try reaching high notes. Any time he began approaching notes above middle C or if he approached a place in his range where he needed to change into an upper register, tension appeared in his voice. Regardless of whether the tension was subconsciously self-induced or not, it was clearly uncomfortable for him to sing in that higher pitch range.

Octave displacement during warm-ups and repertoire singing is a skill many singers learn in choral environments. If an exercise moves into an uncomfortably high range, a singer might continue the vocalise on the same notes an octave down. Octave displacement is especially prevalent in trans choruses and can be a significant challenge for someone going through transition who is relearning how the voice feels in the body. Eli had been learning this skill in his ensemble singing training and private lessons. When he could hear the difference between upper voice parts and lower voice parts, he matched pitch easily within harmonies. He distinguished the disparities in tone color between high and low voices and found himself at home with other low-voice singers. Problems arose, however, when all parts were singing in unison. Delineations between high and low voices became more difficult to distinguish and Eli felt lost in the soup of sound. During a rehearsal once, Eli was able to name that as part of his vocal dysphoria; he was singing the same notes as the "sopranos" and felt uncomfortable, even though he was singing an octave down. At this stage, associations with femininity were fraught with dysphoria and extreme discomfort for him, even in a group voice setting like chorus. Upon discussing his experience and the feeling of vocal dysphoria with the rest of the group, he found that the other members experienced similar feelings at times as well.

As he continued with his training, Eli developed a richer baritone voice quality, and although his voice range did not extend any further down, he enjoyed using it more and gained more confidence. Slowly, more notes in the upper register appeared. This upper range extension could have been due in part to the increased stability in his voice after hormone therapy for over 2 years and to increased comfort and confidence in his voice. He soon realized that pitch was only one of many gender markers in voice and that regardless of what pitch range he was singing in, he still sounded like himself. As his skill and confidence grew, Eli had more nuance and more ways to play with his voice, and pitch became less of a concern.

REGISTRATION

Voice registers are complex interactions of acoustic events, muscle control, depth of vocal fold tissue vibration, resonance, vowel shape, style, and so on. Defining registers of the voice is a debated topic among singing teachers, but it is more useful for the purpose of this text to describe registration events specific to transgender singers. In the broadest terms, consider *chest voice* to be dominated by the thyroarytenoid muscles with deep tissue vibration and shorter vocal fold length, *head voice* to be dominated by the cricothyroid muscles with shallow tissue vibration and elongated vocal folds, and *mixed voice* to be somewhere in between.

Controlled maneuvers between registers require a high level of skill and nuance, as well as flexibility in a healthy vocal instrument. Any number of factors might influence a singer's ability to flawlessly maneuver registers, including breath management, dynamic control, muscle coordination, tension, self-awareness, stress, or general vocal health. A transgender singer faces the same challenges, compounded by aspects of social and medical transition and the added stress of vocal dysphoria, if it is present. A chest binder or waist trainer limits the singer's ability to find stability in the body and breath and can cause tension in the neck, shoulders, or back. Hormone therapy, particularly testosterone hormone therapy, can cause rapid and dramatic changes in vocal fold tissue and muscle mass. Even if a transgender singer was adept at register maneuvers before transition, the skills or mind-sets that ensured that ease may become ineffective or counterintuitive.

Considerations for Low-Voice Trans Masculine Singers

When testosterone enters the body, whether during adolescence or later in life, the voice permanently lowers in pitch (Puts, Gaulin, & Verdolini, 2006). Some trans men or trans masculine individuals decide to undergo testosterone hormone therapy to achieve a lower voice. It was previously assumed that testosterone would provide adequate voice change and that trans men would need very little voice training after beginning hormone therapy, but that may not necessarily be the case (Davies & Goldberg, 2006). Adding testosterone to an adult body does not guarantee that an individual's voice will drop, and it certainly does not guarantee that the individual will be satisfied with their voice.

"Trans guy voice" is a phenomenon that most trans masculine vocalists are familiar with, especially as it relates to testosterone hormone therapy. It describes a small, tense, rough sound that is limited in range and dynamic contrast. A teacher might hear that the voice is limited to either a low pitch range that sounds husky and heavy or a very high pitch range that sounds flute-like and thin, but not much between. There may be abrupt register shifts, accompanied by instability, tension, and even holes where phonation is nearly impossible (Constansis, 2008). Refer to Figure 6–1 in Chapter 6 for more information about voice range changes during hormone therapy.

Balance through register maneuvers requires that the tissue of the vocal folds be supple, supported by expert coordination of the mechanism. A singer who has started testosterone therapy as an adult may experience unwanted stiffness or brittleness that prevents smooth transitions through different registers. Because the vocal folds have increased in mass, but the surrounding laryngeal cartilages have not increased in size, the ability of the vocal folds to vibrate freely could be limited (Constansis, 2008). Additionally, altering the depth of vibration in order to change registration during phonation could be limited because of reduced flexibility. Achieving full chest voice may be a challenge for a singer during hormonal transition, and building the muscle coordination required to maintain consistent voice production takes time. In a body that produces its own testosterone, the length of time for voice change is slow and gradual. When adding testosterone from an outside source, changes in voice range may be sudden, leaving less time for the vocal mechanism to adjust to new physiology (Constansis, 2008).

Exercises to improve flexibility through registration for a singer undergoing testosterone therapy could focus on increasing efficiency of breath, improving medial compression without undo tension, and improving coordination between the thyroarytenoid and cricothyroid muscles. Alternating between registers on the same pitch at different volume levels will help the singer learn to adjust muscle tension, vocal fold stiffness and elongation, lung pressure, and resonance. Onset and staccato exercises help train the muscles used in adduction to adequately close the glottis and will help the singer discover the right amount of lung pressure required for beginning phonation. Semi-occluded vocal tract exercises can be used as a helpful training tool for developing laryngeal muscular coordination (Laukkanen, Titze, Hoffman, & Finnegan, 2008). Additional research for singers during testosterone therapy is needed, specifically focused on registration. Singing teachers are well equipped to guide students through registration adjustments, supported by knowledge of vocal function.

Considerations for High-Voice Trans Feminine Singers

If a singer whose body has produced its own testosterone at some point in life chooses to extend their vocal range upward, different concerns present. Head voice production may be weak or hindered by tension when beginning voice training. Some speech feminization techniques utilize an altered laryngeal position that, if performed improperly, could induce tension in the muscles around the larynx that would inhibit freedom in singing. It may be tempting to ask the student to first discover comfortable vocal production in the lower range and then translate that ease into range extension exercises, but this should only be attempted after discussion about how singing in the low range might feel for the student, psychologically and emotionally. Emotional distress can inhibit a singer's ability, especially if the distress arises from the voice itself.

Exercises to guide a singer toward upper range extension and exhibition of feminine gender markers in that upper range would include cricothyroid strengthening, efficient breath management, and tension release, especially in the base of the tongue. Alternating between chest voice and head voice through interval leaps can increase awareness of the sensation of releasing the thyroarytenoid muscles in favor of the cricothyroid muscles. The "tongue buckle" exercise described by Kozan (2012) encourages efficient vocal production free from tension in the tongue. Singers may have trouble matching pitch when first learning to release tension, and recalibration of the experience of the voice in the body may be a necessary stage in voice training. Semi-occluded vocal tract exercises give the singer immediate aural feedback about breath management and efficient production: absence of any hissing caused by escaping air through a straw could indicate healthy, aligned voice production. As with trans masculine low-voiced singers, teachers are already well equipped to develop pedagogical tools for their students.

NATURAL, AUTHENTIC VOICE

Pitch and registration influence a listener as parts of the tapestry of voice, but they are only parts. Resonance and articulation also contain gender markers that affect gender perception. Maintaining a pitch range that feels congruent with the singer's identity manifests in unique ways for each person. Providing affirmation to the student that it is not necessary to change their pitch range or register to discover a natural, authentic voice builds confidence and trust while the singer develops their instrument. At the same time, teachers can help craft and work toward the goals that are outlined by students through accurate management of expectations and skillful use of exercises.

REFERENCES

Adler, R., Hirsch, S., & Mordaunt, M. (2012). *Voice and communication therapy for the transgender/transsexual client*. San Diego, CA: Plural.

Constansis, A. N. (2008). The changing female-to-male (FTM) voice. *Radical Musicology, 3*, 32 pars.

Davies, S., & Goldberg, J. (2006). *Trans care: Changing speech*. Vancouver, Canada: Trans Care Project.

Kozan, A. (2012). The singing voice. In R. Adler, S. Hirsch, & M. Mordaunt (Eds.), *Voice and communication therapy for the transgender/transsexual client* (pp. 413–458). San Diego, CA: Plural.

Laukkanen, A.-M., Titze, I. R., Hoffman, H., & Finnegan, E. (2008). Effects of a semi-occluded vocal tract on laryngeal muscle activity and glottal adduction in a single female subject. *Folia Phoniatrica et Logopaedica, 60*, 298–311.

Puts, D. A., Gaulin, S. J., & Verdolini, K. (2006). Dominance and the evolution of sexual dimorphism in human voice pitch. *Evolution and Behavior, 27*, 283–296.

Reynolds, H. M. (2014). Social transition. In L. Erickson-Schroth (Ed.), *Trans bodies, trans selves: A resource for the transgender community* (pp. 124–154). New York, NY: Oxford University Press.

Serano, J. (2013). *Excluded: Making feminist and queer movements more inclusive* (pp. 28–29). Berkeley, CA: Seal Press.

8

Resonance and Articulation

Consider that people will talk about the fact that I now "pass" as a woman, but nobody ever asks about how difficult it must have been for me to "pass" as a man before.

—Julia Serano, *Whipping Girl: A Transsexual Woman on Sexism and the Scapegoating of Femininity* (p. 180)

INTRODUCTION

A student who found it difficult to maintain attention on all the different aspects of voice stepped up to the whiteboard during a lesson and drew a tree with several branches and a thick trunk. She labeled the roots as posture, the trunk as breath, and the branches she labeled pitch, register, resonance, phrasing, and articulation. She called her artistic invention The Focus Tree, and it has been a useful tool that allows her to describe different successes and challenges in her voice training and to practice bringing these different elements into alignment. Voice is not a linear instrument; each branch on the tree affects the other branches, and each aspect of voice production is interdependent with each other aspect.

Resonance and articulation, although they are discussed toward the end of the pedagogical section of this text, influence the way people hear gender in voices in significant ways. Some transgender or nonbinary singers may be hesitant to change their singing voices for fear of sounding artificial or somehow "off," because they may not understand which of the gender markers in voice is out of alignment. Teachers who can delineate different aspects of a voice and define parameters for success for their students that are in line with the student's goals, within reasonable expectations and physical limitations of the instrument, equip the singer to continue growing their own Focus Tree and develop their own vocal artistry. This section outlines differences in vocal quality and articulatory patterns between points on the gender spectrum and gives tools for teachers to guide their students to discover personal choices about voice production.

RESONANCE AND GENDER PERCEPTION

Once an initial buzz begins at the vocal folds, it is filtered through the resonance tract consisting of the pharynx, mouth, nose, and lips. Along the way, some harmonics are dampened and some are amplified. The length, shape, and suppleness of the resonance tract determine which harmonics are amplified—it determines the vocal resonances (Titze, 2000a; Vennard, 1968). Changing the distance from the vocal folds to the lips, changing the shape of the vowels, and adjusting the placement of consonants—all of these factors influence how listeners hear the quality of a voice. And naturally, all of these factors influence the perception of gender in a voice.

Chapter 7 discussed the importance of pitch as it relates to gender perception, and it is worth noting the amount of pitch range overlap between voice parts of singers and among speakers. Pitch is an important factor in gender perception of voice, but timbre may play a more influential role than pitch. Pernet and Belin (2012) showed that listeners can categorize gender in voices based on timbre information alone (Pernet & Belin, 2012).

Figure 8–1 shows differences in size and length between larger and smaller vocal instruments. Long, wide resonance tracts with low laryngeal positions tend to produce deeper, darker timbres than short, narrow resonance tracts with slightly higher laryngeal positions (Markova, et al., 2016). Although both voices might sing confidently within the same pitch range, the quality of sound in each instrument could vary dramatically. The listener's brain may automatically categorize the larger instrument as male and the smaller instrument as female (Pernet & Belin, 2012).

For transgender singers whose goals include influencing the listener toward a specifically gendered (or gender-neutral) sound, adjusting the vocal tract through changes in resonance and articulatory patterns can have significant effect. It is important for teachers to be aware of the prevalence of do-it-yourself videos, blogs, and online forums that promote overt manipulation of laryngeal positioning in ways that can induce undue tension and to guide students toward the same goals while ensuring sustainability and healthy vocal function.

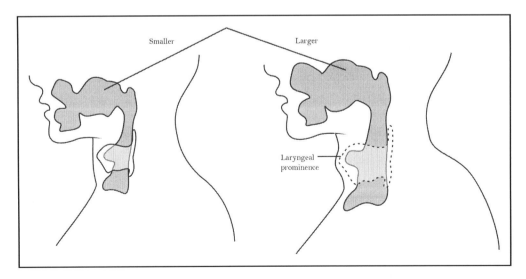

Figure 8–1. Larger and smaller resonance tracts.

Conversely, some singers may be reticent to change the pitch of their voice, even if that is their goal, because they are afraid of sounding artificial. The knowledge they lack is that of aligning the color of the voice with the pitch range. Misgendering still happens for some trans people who change the pitch of their voice either through range extension training or hormone treatment or both, because the quality of the voice is incongruent with the pitch range. Hirsch and Gelfer (2012) state, "Changes in [speaking fundamental frequency] alone may not guarantee a perception of femininity. . . . It is possible there is an inherent 'feminine sound' based on overall vocal tract size and configuration." (Hirsch & Gelfer, 2012, p. 230) Pitch range adjustment on its own may not produce the desired result for the transitioning singer, but in combination with vocal tract adjustment, singers can potentially find a voice that is authentic, natural, and sustainable.

Masculinization of Voice Quality

One of the characteristic features of a masculine-perceived voice is the alignment of resonances produced as a result of a low larynx position. During adolescence in people whose bodies produce testosterone naturally, the larynx grows in size, vocal folds lengthen, and the position of the larynx lowers (Vorperian, et al., 2001). For a trans or nonbinary singer, larynx position can play a significant role in the gender perception of their voice. Lowering the larynx elongates the resonance tract and creates a deeper, broader sound (Markova et al., 2016). Some singers who have been socialized as female may be reluctant or ill-informed about establishing a comfortably low larynx position. Overtly manipulating larynx position can be unsustainable and can cause tension, which may result in harmful compensatory methods and long-term limitations of the whole instrument (Vennard, 1968). Practice patience and gradual change so as not to induce tension or hyperactivity in extralaryngeal muscles.

Changing the position of the tongue in a way that allows the larynx to sit lower may be a safer method, provided that tension is monitored carefully. Figure 8–2 shows a suggested alteration in tongue position for singers working to achieve a deeper, darker sound. The tongue is broad and flat in the back, which in turn broadens the oropharynx and alters the timbre of the voice. Exercises to help achieve this broad, flat tongue should first include methods for tension release. The tongue

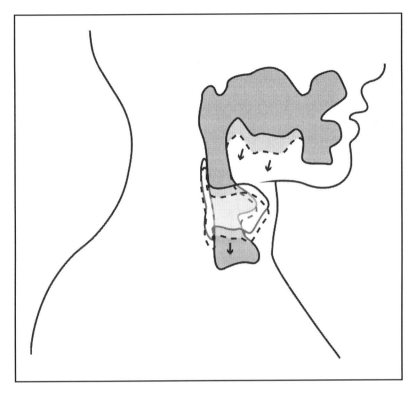

Figure 8–2. Adjustment for masculinization of resonance and articulation.

has complex and very strong muscles, and even indirect changes in laryngeal positioning can be accompanied by chronic tension (LeFevre, 2011). Teachers must keep a close eye and attentive ear for signs of tongue, jaw, or other muscle tension. Exercises that encourage independent movement of the tongue and larynx build strength and flexibility while learning this technique (LeFevre, 2011).

Once the path toward a released tongue is established, students can try altering the color of the voice through vowel modification, which also encourages a lower larynx position and darker timbre. Closed [o] sounds in words such as "bore," "dole," or "whoa" combine sensations of resonance in the mouth with open sounds that encourage a comfortably low larynx position. Replacing sung vowels with [ʌ] as in the words "muppet" or "under" can also help students practice a broad, flat tongue shape. Figure 8–3 shows the opening phrase from "Caro Mio Ben" with the vowels replaced by [ʌ] sounds. Students can explore these adjustments to find a vocal quality that is congruent with how they wish to use their voice and is healthy and sustainable to produce.

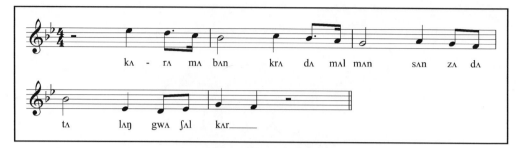

Figure 8–3. Masculinizing vowel exercise, excerpt from "Caro Mio Ben."

Box 8–1. Liam

Liam had received some voice training in choirs and as a (female) musical theater singer but wanted to explore new vocal colors and strengthen his singing voice. As a result of his previous training, his typical larynx position was quite high, which shortened his vocal tract and gave him a characteristically treble voice with a bright color and not much depth.

Liam began learning about the anatomy and physiology of his voice, and that knowledge gave him a great deal of clarity and autonomy with his instrument. It was challenging at first for him to maintain a relaxed larynx position while singing. He had years of training and socialization that led him to believe that a lower larynx was not only undesirable but nearly impossible. He was unhappy with his voice and had disconnected from it, so much so that even significant changes in sound were difficult for him to perceive and integrate.

Over several months, Liam's confidence grew along with familiarity with his instrument. His larynx started to lower and he noticed the rich, full sounds that emerged. He still works to keep his tongue tension in check so that he can sustainably support the vocal quality he wants to create. High pitches are also sometimes troublesome, partly because he feels some dysphoria about that part of his range, which, in turn, affects his technical ability.

Part of the journey has been allowing him to make sounds that didn't emerge from the memory of his old voice, to make sounds that were completely new to him.

In a life where blending in is safer than doing something new, this act of taking up auditory space to make sounds that were, for him, more aligned with his masculinity but were still brand new was exceptionally brave.

Feminization of Voice Quality

Voices that are perceived as feminine have a brighter quality than those perceived as masculine, partially due to shorter resonance tracts (Pernet & Belin, 2012). Shortening the distance from the vocal folds to the lips accentuates upper partials and gives a flutier, lighter sound (Manny, 2014; Vorperian et al., 2001). For trans singers whose bodies naturally produced testosterone at some point in life, achieving a brighter voice quality can be challenging, particularly in combination with a new pitch range and register. It may be helpful to utilize changes in timbre to strengthen voice production in new or previously unused parts of a singer's range. Aligning vocal resonances with sung pitches aids in healthy, sustainable voice production and can be a useful tool in developing a strong head voice, if that is in alignment with the singer's goals and the teacher's reasonable expectations (Titze, 2000b).

The teacher's challenge is to help the student discover ways of achieving a shorter, narrower vocal tract without inducing undue tension such that it limits the singer's technical proficiency. A constricted throat will likely produce a constricted sound, rather than allowing the singer to use their voice freely (Vennard, 1968). To encourage a shorter resonance tract, vowel modification and recalibration of tongue position may be effective with long-term results.

High, forward tongue placement can help to create a brighter, shimmering voice quality. Figure 8–4 shows suggested alterations for tongue position to shorten the resonance tract and amplify high frequencies for a bright sound. Singers can also use vowel modification to achieve this result. The high, forward vowel [i] has been shown to correlate with increased perception of femininity in trans female voices (Hirsch & Gelfer, 2012). In Figure 8–5, the vowels of the first phrase of "Caro Mio Ben" have been replaced with the [i] sound. Utilize this "/i/-ification" of the text to develop new resonance alignment that is more feminine-perceived (Hirsch &Gelfer, 2012).

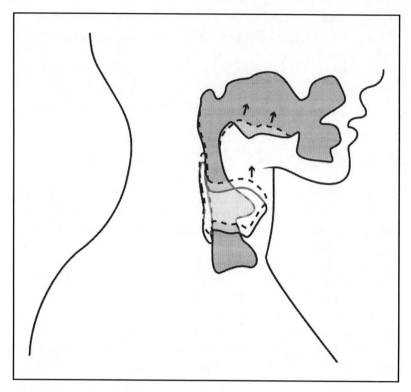

Figure 8–4. Adjustment for feminization of resonance and articulation.

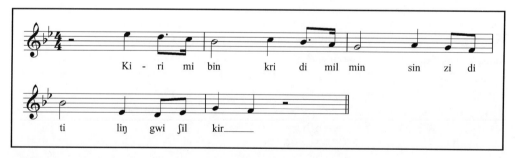

Figure 8–5. Feminizing vowel exercise, excerpt from "Caro Mio Ben."

It might be useful to exaggerate other vowels toward their brighter or more forward counterparts, as shown in Table 8–1. Encouraging a wide lip shape and lifted tongue can alter the resonances of the singer's voice to be more feminine perceived (Manny, 2014).

Table 8–1. Masculinization and Feminization of Vowels

Masculine Perceived	Neutral	Feminine Perceived
ɪ		i
ɛ		e
ɒ	ɑ	a
	ʌ	
	o	
	u	ʊ

Box 8–2. Lorraine

Lorraine is an active singer in several choral ensembles and as a soloist. She has been singing tenor for several years and decided to resume voice lessons once beginning transition, to learn whether a sustainable higher range was a possibility for her. She had been exploring her speaking voice and utilized tools from singing training to aid her in developing speech habits that felt authentic and were healthy. As she started unlocking her upper ranges in singing, some old habits from previous training remained. Namely, the way she maneuvered through middle voice into head voice. Her sound, although in the same pitch ranges as a mezzo-soprano, was dark and broad in a way that did not align with the repertoire she was studying. She was frustrated and described the sound as artificial, even cartoon-like. She also did not have much strength or stamina in the upper range and felt her voice was markedly weak compared to what she was used to.

The muscle memory that Lorraine created to maneuver high notes as a tenor did not always serve her in her new pitch range and was not helping her create the bright, shimmering timbre she wanted. Lorraine also wore body-shaping garments, which at times made it difficult to manage new techniques, and some body dysphoria made it difficult for her to focus on and identify sensations of

> *her voice in her body. Upon exploring changes in her resonance tract that would enhance and add color to the sound, she discovered more harmonic richness and in turn more intensity and strength in her head voice. She learned that she could create different colors in her upper register by allowing her tongue to be high and forward and by spreading her lips. Additionally, adding proprioceptive tools gave her more of a feeling of control as she learned to modify her vowels differently in different parts of her new range. She learned quickly how to use her natural gesticulations when singing to help guide her attention toward resonance and remarked that she finally understood why people "sing with their hands."*

ARTICULATION

Differences in articulation between genders have long been the subject of study in voice and speech. One common, and perhaps oversimplified, conclusion is that women tend to use more socially favored patterns—more "correct" patterns—of articulation than men (Boonin, 2012). It has been posited that people socialized as female learned to create and practice precise or more favored articulation as a means to achieve social status and that feminine-perceived articulation patterns tend to be more precise than masculine-perceived articulation patterns (Boonin, 2012).

In singing, proficient and easily intelligible diction is important, regardless of gender identity or vocal gender presentation. The notion that feminine-identified/presenting singers and masculine-identified/presenting singers should use more or less precise diction to influence listeners to hear a particular gender in voice is probably more useful in speech than in singing. A different approach might be to consider forward articulation and back articulation, rather than precise or imprecise, with additional consideration given to the pressurization of consonants.

Hirsch and Gelfer (2012) suggest using *acoustic assumptions*, or "why the voice sounds a certain way under certain conditions" to help the student make desired changes to articulatory patterns. For example, voiced consonants are darker than their unvoiced counterparts; pressurized consonants are also darker. When creating an [f] sound, if the bottom lip is tucked underneath the top teeth, there is more pressure inside the mouth before the release of the [f] sound. If the bottom lip rests just in front of the top teeth, however, [f] is more fluid and airy with little or no pressure inside the mouth. The former, being darker, is perceived as more masculine; the latter, being brighter, is perceived as more feminine (Hirsch & Gelfer, 2012).

Exercises for the singer can include building awareness of acoustic assumptions and habitual patterns, through transcription of diction and self-evaluation of tongue, lip, and mouth position. If the student's goals include a darker or more masculine-perceived voice, exercises to induce more pressurized consonants and darker vowel sounds could be helpful. For singers whose goals include a brighter or more feminine-perceived voice, exercises might include lightening consonants. A lighter touch, with the sounds rolling off the tip of the tongue, may influence the listener to hear a more feminine voice than slow articulation that resides more at the back of the tongue (Boonin, 2012).

ALL THE BRANCHES OF THE FOCUS TREE

Singing is a complex process involving many different aspects of technique that are interdependent. Each branch of The Focus Tree is most successfully executed when all the other branches are in alignment as well. Singing teachers are uniquely gifted at finding ways to bring students' attention to a particular aspect of technique while balancing all the others and building skills in coordination. Many of the considerations for gender perception discussed in these chapters already reside within the singing teacher's skillset but are likely used in a different way or to produce a different result.

Developing efficient breath management and body alignment is at the center of singing technique, and teachers are already equipped to help students learn about respiration; the new challenge may be guiding a student who wears a body-shaping garment while being mindful and respectful of potential body dysphoria. Teachers already have tools to help students develop healthy, sustainable phonation through the entire pitch range and through different registers, although the challenge for the teacher of a transgender or nonbinary singer will be evaluating the singer's goals and designing processes to support those goals with reasonable expectations. Much of the literature on voice technique encourages an open, relaxed throat and clear diction; the difference for trans singers is in finding vocal tract positions and articulatory habits that align with a desired outcome as it relates to gender perception. Singing teachers are well equipped to utilize teaching tools, knowledge, experience, and expertise, informed by cultural competence and led by the student.

REFERENCES

Boonin, J. (2012). Articulation. In R. Adler, S. Hirsch, & M. Mordaunt (Eds.), *Voice and communication therapy for the transgender/transsexual client: A comprehensive clinical guide* (pp. 249–261). San Diego, CA: Plural.

Hirsch, S. & Gelfer, M. P. (2012). Resonance. In R. Adler, S. Hirsch, & M. Mordaunt (Eds.), *Voice and communication therapy for the transgender/transsexual client: A comprehensive clinical guide* (pp. 225–247). San Diego, CA: Plural.

LeFevre, C. (2011, November/December). Tongue management. *Journal of Singing, 68*(2), 157–162.

Manny, E. (2014). *The male-to-female transgender voice: Most salient voice parameters in perceived gender identification.* Boston, MA: Northeastern University.

Markova, D., Richer, L., Pangelinan, M., Schwartz, D. H., Leonard, G., Perron, M., . . . Tomas, P. (2016). Age- and sex-related variations in vocal-tract morphology and voice acoustics during adolescence. *Hormones and Behavior, 81*, 84–96.

Pernet, C. R., & Belin, P. (2012). The role of pitch and timbre in voice gender categorization. *Frontiers in Psychology, 3*(23), 1–11.

Serano, Julia. (2016). *Whipping girl, a transsexual woman on sexism and the scapegoating of femininity.* Berkeley, CA: Seal Press.

Titze, I. R. (2000a). The source-filter theory of vowels. In I. R. Titze (Ed.), *Principles of voice production* (pp. 149–184). Iowa City, IA: National Center for Voice and Speech.

Titze, I. R. (2000b). Vocal fold oscillation. In I. R. Titze (Ed.), *Principles of voice production* (pp. 87–122). Iowa City, IA: National Center for Voice and Speech.

Vennard, W. (1968). Resonance. In W. Vennard (Ed.), *Singing the mechanism and the technic* (pp. 101–110). Los Angeles, CA: Carl Fisher.

Vorperian, H. K., Wang, S., Schimek, E. M., Durtschi, R. B., Kent, R. D., Gentry, L. R., & Chung, M. K. (2001). Developmental sexual dimorphism of the oral and pharyngeal positions of the vocal tract: An imaging study. *Journal of Speech, Language, and Hearing Research, 54*, 995–1010.

Voice Health for Transgender Singers

According to my voice teacher, the only way I could find my female voice was to realize that there was no difference between what I was and what I wanted to be. The voice of my future wasn't something to strive for, it was something to relax into . . . I would find my voice by speaking as myself.

—Joy Ladin, *Gender Outlaws: The Next Generation* (p. 254)

INTRODUCTION

All singers should have an understanding of the basic mechanism and function of their voices and ensure adequate vocal hygiene for a healthy instrument. Training such a detailed and complex instrument takes dedication and experience, and also self-awareness of what is "normal" from day to day. When something goes wrong, singers sometimes feel bewildered and helpless because the voice is not like any other instrument—there are no strings to replace, the pipes cannot be removed and cleaned or examined on their own, and it may be difficult or impossible to point to the problem from outside the instrument. Because the voice exists as a whole and it is challenging (and potentially counterintuitive) to separate it into its parts in order to determine the cause of the discomfort or dysfunction, regular maintenance and commitment to intimate knowledge of the instrument by the vocalist is a must.

The voice can sometimes feel like an abstract or intangible part of the body that seems to work of its own accord whether given explicit instructions or not. For a trans singer who experiences vocal dysphoria and/or body dysphoria, that feeling of disconnection can be strong. In *Gender Outlaws: The Next Generation* (2010), Joy Ladin describes voice training:

> I no longer had anything that could be called "my voice." . . . I could feel the air moving in my throat, my mouth, in the cavities of my head as I spoke; I could shape it, direct it, increase and decrease amplitude, breathiness, resonance. The result was a new voice, or rather a series of new voices. . . . These voices were strained, unreliable, and required constant thought and effort . . . I couldn't shake the sense that my voice was a caricature." (Ladin, 2010, p. 253)

Maintaining constant awareness of voice use to avoid straining the voice during vocal transition, however that manifests for the singer, can help ensure that the singer feels connected to their voice and that it is well cared for. This section outlines some of the basics of vocal hygiene as well as some specific voice health challenges that transgender and nonbinary singers may face.

VOCAL HYGIENE

Vocal hygiene refers to daily care and maintenance of the vocal instrument, including proper hydration, knowledge of medications and their effects on the voice, a voice-healthy diet, and adequate voice recovery. Maintaining a practice of daily vocal hygiene builds the singer's awareness of their instrument, noticing subtle changes from day to day or through hormonal cycles, and when significant changes occur.

Hydration During Medical Transition

Adequate hydration is vital for singers, to help maintain effective lubrication of the vocal folds. Without adequate hydration, the mucus that coats the vocal folds becomes thick and tacky, which, in turn, does very little to dissipate heat caused by friction from vibration. In an attempt to cool the tissue, the vocal folds swell, causing inefficient vibration and increased phonation threshold pressure (Gates, 2013; Sivasankar & Leydon, 2010). Swollen vocal folds can present problems for the singer and may lead to more concerning vocal damage (Sivasankar & Leydon, 2010). This is especially true for singers exploring new voice ranges and techniques, since the exercises and vocal demands of a transitioning singer may be more rigorous in some ways than for cisgender signers.

Trans individuals receive a myriad of medications, not least of which is hormone therapy of some kind, if they choose to utilize hormone therapy as part of medical transition. Testosterone and estrogen drugs usually contain some kind of diuretic, and singers taking these medications should increase their water intake to maintain adequate hydration and vocal fold lubrication (National Center for Voice and Speech, 2015). Some trans people also choose to take medication for mental health, digestive health, or seasonal allergies. Antidepressants or antianxiety medications, allergy medications, and heartburn medications all have similar drying effects and should be counteracted with increased hydration (National Center for Voice and Speech, 2015).

Anti-inflammatory medications and anticoagulants such as ibuprofen, aspirin, and naproxen (Excedrin) should be avoided when possible. These drugs thin the blood, which can increase the risk of vocal fold hemorrhage (National Center for Voice and Speech, 2015). A trans singer combatting physical discomfort from body-shaping garments, for example, may find themselves in need of an analgesic. Acetaminophen (Tylenol) serves this purpose better for a singer than aspirin or ibuprofen (Gates, 2013; Titze & Abbott, 2012). Conversations about medications with students can begin at the first lesson and should continue throughout the student's length of study, with particular attention to adequate hydration.

Box 9–1. Bailey

When Bailey began voice training, she complained of constant dryness in her throat and mouth, and cleared her throat often. At the time, she was engaged in hormone replacement therapy; she took estrogen supplements and androgen blockers, both diuretics that can cause drying and present challenges for maintaining adequate hydration. The mucus in Bailey's body was gummy and heavy, which made voice production challenging for her. In addition to challenges for voice health presented by her hormone therapy, Bailey also had acid reflux. Compounded by her active weekend lifestyle, digestive troubles presented voice health problems as well.

Through the process of her medical transition, Bailey and her endocrinologist eventually adjusted her hormone treatment levels, which gave her an opportunity to enjoy more adequate hydration. She also decided to start medication for her reflux and change her diet, significantly reducing the thick, sticky mucus that plagued her and caused her to clear her throat so often. As her body adjusted to these positive changes in vocal hygiene, she also fought the urge to clear her throat and eventually kicked the habit. Her vocal stamina increased, as did her enjoyment in lessons because her instrument could keep up with her excitement and eagerness to learn.

Nutrition

For all singers, teachers typically recommend a voice-healthy diet. Different types of foods produce different digestive responses, which sometimes manifest in the ways the body produces mucus. Dairy products, high-acid fruits, and sugar all create a digestive response that produces thick, viscous mucus throughout the body, including the larynx (Gates, 2013). Greasy and spicy foods can also cause heartburn and acid reflux, a common problem for singers. A diet rich in protein and fiber, complex carbohydrates, and fruits and vegetables that have high water content is ideal for most singers (Gates, 2013).

Voice Recovery and Cool-Downs

Singing is an athletic activity; it requires virtuosic control of a nonlinear biomechanical system, and physical and psychological stamina (Titze, 2000). Constant vibration of the vocal folds causes friction and wear on the vocal fold tissue, and training new techniques can cause fatigue in the laryngeal muscles (Gates, 2013). Just as with any athlete, singers must schedule time for rest and recuperation. As trans singers develop new singing techniques, they may be taxing the vocal muscles and tissues more than in previous voice study and should schedule extra time during the initial training periods to rest and recover after voice lessons, coachings, rehearsals, performances, and other heavy vocal loading periods. A cool-down regimen that includes semi-occluded vocal tract techniques such as straw phonation, humming, lip buzzes, or tongue trills benefits vocal health (Titze & Abbott, 2012; Verdolini Abbott et al., 2012).

POTENTIAL FOR VOICE DISORDERS

Only a medical doctor can diagnose a voice disorder, and trans students benefit from the support of a voice team consisting of an otolaryngologist, speech pathologist, and singing teacher (World Professional Association for Transgender Health, 2017). Singing training, particularly singing training through transition, can put a heavy load on the voice, especially when the singer simultaneously works to alleviate vocal or other forms of dysphoria in daily life. Singers and teachers understand the role that emotional and psychological states can have in allowing or limiting vocal freedom and ability to acquire new singing skills. Keep a close eye on voice function over time, and if changes occur that impede vocal growth, seek the guidance of fellow voice care professionals.

Consistent hoarseness or raspy voice or inability to access high registers can be signs of vocal fold edema, which can lead to more complex vocal issues (Gates, 2013). Semi-occlusion exercises have been proven to reduce vocal fold swelling and could be used as both warm-up and cool-down exercises for singing students (Verdolini Abbott et al., 2012). If symptoms persist, it is recommended that the student visit a voice-specialized speech pathologist, laryngologist, and/or singing voice specialist for further direction. There is a growing number of voice care professionals who are trans-competent and educated in the specific voice needs of trans individuals.

While encouraging the singer to explore changes in phonatory patterns, laryngeal positioning, tongue carriage, and lip shape, it is imperative to ensure that the laryngeal mechanism can support these changes. Chronic tension in the muscles outside the larynx or near the muscle groups responsible for phonation may appear as compensatory methods for inability to maintain easy, relaxed phonation (Gates, 2013). If the student begins to experience vocal fatigue, laryngeal muscle fatigue, inflexibility, breaks in phonation, or pain in the back of the neck, it may be time to readdress healthy voice techniques and help the student create vocal habits that encourage free and easy voice production. If problems persist, the student may benefit from a visit to a speech pathologist.

It is not uncommon for trans students to begin voice lessons having already experimented with different ways of speaking or singing in order to align their voice with their gender, alleviate vocal dysphoria, or influence others to perceive their voice as more masculine or more feminine. Sometimes self-guided vocal work can create or reinforce inefficient voice habits, and these must be addressed and resolved just like with any other singing student. The unique challenge for teachers of trans singers, especially singers who are exploring new ranges or voice parts, is to continually encourage and discover natural, authentic voice production and realistically support the student's goals. If any uncertainty arises about the vocal health of a student, refer to a fellow voice care professional such as a singing voice specialist, voice-specialized speech pathologist, and/or laryngologist.

DEVELOPING PRACTICE ROUTINES

Just as for all singers, a stable practice routine encourages healthy voice use and efficient implementation of new singing techniques. Refer to Appendix 3 for a sample routine. Some trans singers may experience vocal dysphoria; the sound of their voice seems disconnected with their own self-identity. They may feel discouraged to sing through their entire vocal range or attempt new techniques that heighten their feelings of dysphoria. It is important to continue open dialogue about the student's comfort level in exploring their whole vocal instrument while supporting the goals that teacher and student have agreed upon together. Trans students may need to create a practice schedule during off-peak practice times so that they can explore their instrument without fear of being overheard, judged, or blatantly misgendered by peers or other teachers, until their confidence is bolstered. Maintaining a regular practice routine that reinforces healthy singing habits is important in helping to build confidence and competence, just as with any other singer.

VOICE FEMINIZATION SURGERY

Some transgender women or trans feminine people elect to undergo vocal feminization surgery, which involves changing the structure of the larynx so that the voice sounds more feminine perceived. Below are brief descriptions of types of voice feminization surgeries. Only a surgeon can make medical recommendations for these types of procedures; results for singers are not well documented, however, and a trans singer considering voice feminization surgery would benefit from the support of a complete voice care team, including the singing teacher.

Cricothyroid Approximation (CTA)

Head voice is dominated by the cricothyroid muscles, and this type of voice feminization surgery raises the pitch and helps disengage the thyroarytenoid muscles. Figure 9–1 illustrates a form of cricothyroid approximation surgery.

> Contraction of this muscle brings the thyroid cartilage and cricoid cartilage into approximation in the anterior midline,

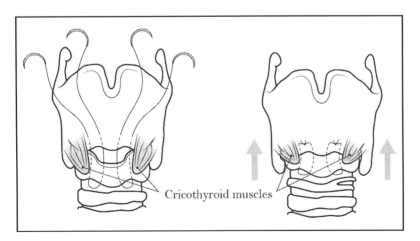

Figure 9–1. Cricothyroid approximation. The thyroid and cricoid cartilages are brought together and fixed or fused.

so CTA surgery effectively sutures the cricothyroid muscle into a permanent position of contraction, although the degree is variable. . . . The surgery then doesn't change speech patterns, intensity, resonance or inflection characteristics of the male voice into a female pattern, rather when successful, it limits the voice to the upper range. This can be a desirable limitation by relieving the effort of always trying to keep the voice up in falsetto. It also generally prevents an inadvertent drop into a deeper voice at an inopportune moment. (Thomas, 2017a, para. 1)

Thyrohyoid Elevation

As discussed in Chapter 8, shorter vocal tracts tend to produce more feminine-perceived sound. This type of surgery is meant to elevate the larynx for a shortened resonance tract. Figure 9–2 illustrates a form of thyrohyoid elevation surgery.

"The thyroid cartilage . . . is exposed and the top portion removed. Holes are placed in the thyroid cartilage and in the hyoid bone and when tightened, the voice box is raised higher in the neck." (Thomas, 2017b, Procedure section, para. 2)

Anterior Glottoplasty

This surgery method shortens the vibrating length of the vocal folds by suturing or webbing together the anterior (front)

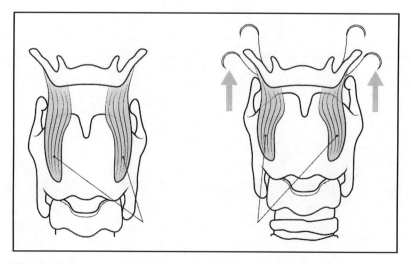

Figure 9–2. Thyrohyoid elevation. The thyroid cartilage is raised to meet the hyoid bone above it, lifting the larynx and shortening the vocal tract.

portion. Figures 9–3A and 9–3B illustrate two different types of this surgery.

"One-third portion of vocal fold membrane and internal tissue [is removed], and then suturing them out tight with permanent suture material using the micro instruments" (Yeson Voice Center, 2018, para. 2).

"Webbing of the anterior portion of the vocal cords is a surgery designed to raise the comfortable speaking pitch by shortening the vibrating length of the vocal cords" (Thomas, 2017c, para. 1)

Feminization Laryngoplasty (FemLar)

FemLar is a complex surgery in which the thyroid cartilage is reduced and the anterior portion of the vocal folds is removed, accompanied by thyrohyoid elevation. The goal is to raise the speaking fundamental frequency and shorten the resonance tract for a brighter voice quality.

> Feminization laryngoplasty is a procedure removing the anterior thyroid cartilage, collapsing the diameter of the larynx as well as shortening and tensioning the vocal folds to raise the pitch. . . . One aspect of the procedure, thyrohyoid approximation (introduced in 2006 to alter resonance), did not affect pitch. Feminization laryngoplasty successfully increased the comfortable fundamental frequency of speech and removed

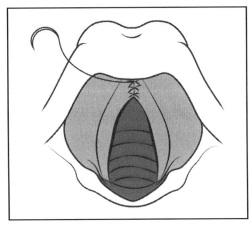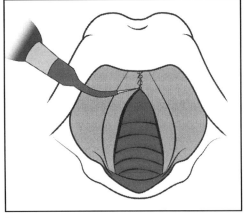

A **B**

Figure 9–3. A. Anterior glottoplasty: suture. The anterior portion of the vocal folds is trimmed and sutured together, shortening the vibrating length and raising the pitch of the voice. **B.** Anterior glottoplasy: laser. The covering of the anterior portion of the vocal folds is removed with a laser.

the lowest notes from the patient's vocal range. It does not typically raise the upper limits of the vocal range. (Thomas & MacMillan, 2013, Abstract section)

RECOMMENDED READING

Bastian Medical Media. (2017a, January 1). *Voice & other larynx disorders*. Retrieved from https://laryngopedia.com/disorders/voice-larynx-disorders/

Bastien Medical Media. (2017b, January 1). *Muscle tension dysphonia*. Retrieved from https://laryngopedia.com/muscular-tension-dysphonia/

Johns, M. M. (2003, December). Update on the etiology, diagnosis, and treatment of vocal fold nodules, polyps, and cysts. *Current Opinion in Otolaryngology & Head and Neck Surgery, 11*(6), 456–461.

Popkin, B. M., D'Anci, K., & Rosenberg, I. H. (2010). Water, hydration, and health. *Nutrition Reviews, 68*(8), 439–458.

REFERENCES

Gates, R. (2013). *The owner's manual to the voice: A guide for singers and professional voice users.* New York, NY: Oxford University Press.

Ladin, J. (2010). The voice. In K. Bornstein & S. B. Bergman (Eds.), *Gender outlaws: The next generation* (pp. 247–254). Berkeley, CA: Seal Press.

National Center for Voice and Speech. (2015, January 1). *Check your meds: Do they affect your voice?* Retrieved from http://www.ncvs.org/rx.html

Sivasankar, M., & Leydon, C. (2010). The role of hydration in vocal fold physiology. *Current Opinion in Otolaryngology & Head and Neck Surgery, 18*(3), 171–175.

Thomas, J. P. (2017a). *Cricothyroid approximation.* Retrieved from https://www.voicedoctor.net/surgery/Pitch/Cricothyroid-approximation

Thomas, J. P. (2017b). *Thyrohyoid elevation.* Retrieved from https://www.voicedoctor.net/surgery/pitch/thyrohyoid-elevation

Thomas, J. P. (2017c). *Web glottoplasty.* Retrieved from https://www.voicedoctor.net/surgery/pitch/web-glottoplasty

Thomas, J. P., & MacMillan, C. (2013). Feminization laryngoplasty: Assessment of surgical pitch elevation. *European Archives of Oto-Rhino-Laryngology, 270*(10), 2695–2700.

Titze, I. (2000). *Principles of voice production.* Iowa City, IA: National Center for Voice and Speech.

Titze, I. R., & Abbott, K. V. (2012). *Vocology: The science and practice of voice habilitation*. Salt Lake City, UT: National Center for Voice and Speech.

Verdolini Abbott, K., Li, N., L., Branski, R., Rosen, C., Grillo, E., Steinhauer, K., . . . Hebda, P. A. (2012). Vocal exercises may attenuate acute vocal fold inflammation. *Journal of Voice, 26*(6), 814.e1–814.e13.

World Professional Association for Transgender Health (WPATH). (2017, January 1). *Standards of care for the health of transsexual, transgender, and gender nonconforming people Version 7.* Retrieved from https://s3.amazonaws.com/amo_hub_content/Association140/files/Standards%20of%20Care%20V7%20-%202011%20WPATH%20(2)(1).pdf

Yeson Voice Center. (2018). *Vocal folds shortening/retrodisplacement of anterior commissure.* Retrieved from http://www.yesonvc.net/page/2_4_1.php

PART THREE

The Experience

CHAPTER
10

Trans Singers
on Singing

INTRODUCTION

As much as this text hopes to outline pedagogical consider-ations for transgender and gender nonconforming singers, its chief function is to bridge theories and clinical studies with practical application and personal connection. Brief narra-tives and encounters distributed through the chapters give examples of some of the most significant moments that trans singers encounter along their voice education journeys. The responsibility of the teacher lies in absorbing and connect-ing to those moments so that students reap the benefits of trans-competency in the voice studio, classroom, rehearsal, audition, or performance. There is an inherent power dynamic between trans people and those who research the experiences of trans people. Often, the research does not directly benefit the people about whom the research is being performed. In talking about training trans singes, it is imperative to amplify the experiences and voices of trans people, rather than allow any of this discussion to remain theoretical. These interviews do not alleviate that dynamic between researcher and subject, nor are they meant to. They are meant to spur conversation, because the best way to learn is to listen.

The singers featured in these interviews range in age, gender identity, ethnicity, professional performance level, and personality across a wide spectrum of experiences. Between them, however, some common themes arise. For each of these singers, there have been phases of life during which teachers and trusted members of their cultural circles have told them to change the way they use their voice because it didn't fit into the expected gender norms. There is anxiety around being "clocked"—more specifically, anxiety about being abandoned by friends and loved ones upon discovering their trans iden-tity. And these singers are constantly carving out authenticity for themselves, dissolving the barriers that kept them from freely expressing their vocal artistry. They have experienced a complex journey toward reclaiming their identities as sing-ers and as people, and we are deeply honored and grateful to share their stories.

JT

JT is a composition, music theory, aural skills, and musician-ship professor at a university; he is also a composer of contem-porary classical music. As a fellow educator and professional musician, he views his voice as an instrument that requires care, curiosity, patience, and dedication just like any other. As a student, he has always been open about his process, willing to try new things and make mistakes (or bizarre new sounds), and actively engages in the partnership of voice lessons. His grounded wisdom and calm, lighthearted demeanor allow him to experiment and grow without harsh self-judgment or apprehension.

In this interview, he talks about his relationship to his voice from high school through adulthood and how it feels to finally begin the path of hormonal transition as a singer. He also talks about compassion as an element of cultural competence as well as the importance of technical expertise for teachers of transgender singers.

Int: indicates the interviewers

JT: indicates the student's response.

Int: Could you start by talking a little about your voice life and your journey as a singer?

JT: I have always sung, and in traditional singing spaces like choirs and private lessons in high school I always felt sort of out of place, particularly with the repertoire. I was uncomfortable with the rep I was singing in voice lessons, and what it meant to be a soprano. And the stuff sopranos sing about, the acting part, I didn't know what it was about it, but I just thought, "I don't think I can do that." But singing is as big of a part of my identity as my gender and I don't think I realized I had vocal dysphoria, really until I started taking lessons as an adult.

Int: Really?

JT: Yeah.

Int: Can you say more about that?

JT: I didn't ever perform a whole lot as a soloist, as a singer, and was a little adverse to that, but I performed in choir. Whenever I heard my voice recorded it would just feel foreign, like it wasn't mine. I think speaking also, like I didn't ever really speak in a very healthy way and I was trying to speak in a lower range than was natural and I was letting my voice fall back in my throat. And I sought out lessons—I can't even remember, I think I was just beginning to identify as male. There was a year before that where I was calling myself gender queer and just coming to terms with everything and figuring it out. And with pronouns, there was a period where I wasn't ready to be "he" or comfortable with "she," but I never felt like a "they" either.

Int: Certainly, there was some trepidation or nervousness in the beginning, and it was clear that you were writing a new and very important chapter of your life.

JT: Yeah, I was beginning to think about transitioning but it scared me to mess with my voice and that was, for a long time, the biggest reason that I didn't want to start hormone therapy. Over the course of studying, I started to realize that I wanted my voice to be different. That became a big reason to go on hormone therapy.

Int: It has been an honor to be part of that conversation with you.

JT: I'm grateful to you—it was helpful to consult with you.

Int: When you started lessons, there was a sense of disconnection from the rep that had been assigned to you in the past, but then eventually you made your way back to classical singing. And then, of course, you debuted as Tamino last spring, which was amazing! What was that like, to go from somewhat of a distaste for classical singing to having the lead in *The Magic Flute*?

JT: Aside from exercises, the most rep I've done has been pop. I think I had an association with classical singing as just being uncomfortable from high school or whatever, and I don't think I was doing it very well. I had a lot of immediate tension even if I thought I was singing classical music. Especially with solo rep.

Int: Do you think that comes from feeling dysphoric about your voice, from not liking the genre, or both?

JT: Probably vocal dysphoria because it was especially true above a certain register, and I love classical music but I have a different relationship with it, performing it as a singer than listening to it, or composing classical contemporary music or anything else. Maybe because my life is in the classical music world, I'd probably rather sing pop music. Or if I was going to sing "classical music" it would be contemporary classical music and that's what I see for myself eventually, on the other side of the change, is to sing some of my own music, which is informed heavily by popular music as well as the classical tradition, but it doesn't sound like older rep. So much of classical rep carries this heteronormative, gender-normative baggage. I see it as a way to be free from that maybe.

Int: You mean performing your own compositions, that's how you find freedom?

JT: Yeah. But it was fun singing Tamino, and it has been fun to come back to classical music with a new relationship to it.

Int: Can you say more about that? What do you think were some of the technical challenges, and what were some of the personal challenges in taking on that role?

JT: The technical challenges at that point—I think the lowest notes were still a stretch and I wanted them fuller and stronger probably, and that was before T. And if I were to really do that expertly I would probably need to be in that world more and put more time into how I do it. I was doing that for fun, but as a perfectionist generally, it just sort of felt like I knew I could do it better, but I was happy.

Int: You blew everyone away! It was gorgeous, so impressive.

JT: Well thank you! What was really fun about that whole experience or, important for me about it, was more the acting than the singing, actually. Just getting to play a guy was a big deal and it felt really good and it was easy and everybody was very accepting, which helped a lot. It didn't occur to anyone that I shouldn't be in that role that I could tell. It was fun.

Int: What was it like to play a straight guy? *The Magic Flute* **is so steeped in heteronormativity and bizarre gender and relationship stereotypes.**

JT: Yeah! Like Papageno and the whole "let's have little a Papageno" thing, and Tamino and it's—yeah, it's ridiculous. It was weird, and it was weird to realize that that was probably my first experience singing as—well, I don't know what I would call myself anymore, as a nonstraight guy—but as a guy. It was the first time I realized that that could be weird and not fit, although it was a much better fit than being a princess that gets rescued—

Int: Oh my, yeah—

JT: It fit better than that, but it made me think about all the gay male opera singers out there and how they cope with that all the time. But even being attracted to women as well as men now, I wouldn't ever want my relationship dynamic to resemble that in any way. But, I don't know, it was fun. It was fun being alpha male leading the other guy around the forest and there are things that felt more right, I guess.

Int: How do you think that impacted your identity as a singer?

JT: I don't know if I'm there yet. I don't know if I know what that identity is yet. I think it just sort of opened it up, or sent a message that it could be anything.

Int: That's exciting! Would you be willing to talk a little bit about your transition and how some of the different aspects of medical transition have affected your voice?

JT: Sure. As of now, so far and I'm probably just about at 4 months on T, I mean it's mainly just that my voice itself is changing. It started with maybe a couple months in or 6 weeks in, I still had my full range but the top notes started to feel like they needed more strength to be produced and it all just kind of started feeling different. And now we're definitely in a weird place, that I guess I'm going to be in for a while. I've read some of the research and have some understanding of what's actually happening. I'm gaining low range and I'm gaining comfort and strength down there, although it's still thinner than a cis male singer's voice in that register.

Int: On the bottom you mean?

JT: Yeah. I was singing with my dad last weekend when he was here, which was kind of interesting.

Int: It's interesting too to think about how pitch-matching and octave displacement navigation is changing. Can you talk about that?

JT: Yeah, that's been interesting as well. My career is teaching musicianship and teaching theory among other things, and I've always been super good at finding a pitch really quickly. Now, it's as if sometimes it's hard to find my comfortable range. If I'm trying to sing along with something that's within a fifth or sixth or seventh below middle C sometimes I'll miss, or if I'm singing along with something that is an octave above that, it's kind of difficult to find an octave down. I'll try singing along and it won't really work and I'll try to go down to the lower octave but then actually go down two octaves. I have to recalibrate and figure out where my comfortable range actually sits, because I'm expecting it to be low, I guess.

Int: Right, and what "low" feels like in your body now is different.

JT: Yeah, and it's like, I need to go low but I overshoot where I need to go, and then I have to come back up. I know sometimes if I'm teaching, I tend to go back and forth between speaking and singing pretty quickly and that's getting a little difficult, that doesn't always work anymore. If I need to talk about something in my musicianship class and then demonstrate it, I don't always aim correctly. Which is fine, it's not a big problem, but that's what's happening.

Int: Just as a nugget of encouragement it's important to remember that if you're comparing your voice to someone else's, like your dad's, that person probably has had more than 4 months to figure that out.

JT: No it's funny, his range and mine are actually sort of similar right now, which is funny. It's almost like we're both in a somewhat limited, baritone-ish range right now and we're trying to figure out who should sing melody and who should sing harmony, and neither way works super well.

Int: Really? That's new! And you and your dad have been singing together forever, right?

JT: Yeah we have. I wondered what it would be like for him. He actually was the one who pulled out the guitar and wanted to sing together and he handled it very well.

Int: Way to go, dad! So related to medical transition, if you're comfortable talking about it, what has it been like after top surgery, not having to wear a binder all the time, especially while singing?

JT: That definitely made a big difference, I mean I know it's common sense that wearing a binder sucks for singing. For me, I'm not sure it was as true. I never wore the tightest binder in the world, but it definitely has changed my posture and the way I carry myself to not be wearing it. It's almost hard to remember. I just know everything got better, and it's definitely easier to breathe and feel free singing.

Int: That's great! In terms of inhabiting your voice as it's changing, have you noticed any changes in your body that make it different, or easier, or harder in terms of embodying a more "masculine" voice?

JT: I don't know. Maybe. I know as my voice gets lower and I'm more comfortable in a lower register, I feel more comfortable and more confident. In terms of physicality, it's hard to know because I was weight-training a lot before starting HRT so I think I'm getting bigger and broader and everything but I'm not sure how much of that is due to testosterone and how big a difference there's been with that specifically in the last 4 months. And I'm also on this really low dose, so I think it's probably very gradually better and better but I can't really tell.

Int: You've been so patient, and it must be hard to just come into this as an adult. Did you have to cope with feelings of discomfort when you were in high school?

JT: I quit voice lessons my senior year. I was playing the trombone also and chose to do that for college. I don't know, maybe that's why I picked the trombone. I think it's funny thinking back on it. I didn't always get along with the choral director super well because I was kind of sharper on some of the musicianship stuff, but I was also maybe feeling some annoyance around singing soprano. So it's hard to separate all of that, and I just started spending more of my time on instrumental music. It always felt good to sing, but knowing that I was singing high didn't feel good, and hearing my voice was never good, and solo rep was usually not going to bring out the best in me. Singing something in Latin that I didn't understand, that wasn't about anything physical, like some really cerebral piece with a bunch of guys and girls was fine, though.

Int: What were some of the more challenging rep choices?

JT: I did the 24 Italian songs and arias, which aren't even necessarily gender specific. I had other stuff, too. "It Was a Lover and His Lass" was rough. I think we were doing some Faure pieces and those are beautiful and I love those, but they didn't feel good. And now thinking about it, it wasn't even that the songs had to be gender specific from a female point of view, but if they were, I was especially uncomfortable. But I don't know, I sang the "Little Mermaid" for fun like everybody else, and enjoyed that. It was always kind of a caricature. And I'll probably go back to Mariah Carey after the change, too.

Int: Can you talk a little bit about when and why you started voice lessons? What were some things that made a positive impact on your ability to find more freedom and authenticity in your voice?

JT: Hmm. I don't know . . . because it felt good to sing. I'm remembering starting lessons again and I came to it wanting to lower my speaking voice without changing my singing voice, and over time I realized that I wanted to change that too.

Int: Were there things that clicked for you that made you realize that?

JT: There were probably times when we were exploring upper registers and I was more self-aware than I was when I was younger, enough to be like, "I hate this."

Int: Right, you had ways to categorize and figure out why it was uncomfortable.

JT: Yeah and I think there was one voice lesson that we tried a pants role song or something, it was some classical piece in a soprano register and I was just like, "I hate singing this and I don't want to do it."

Int: Yep. There was both a sense that it was really beautiful music, and like, "please don't make me do this."

JT: I was noticing that I wanted to sing it better because it was beautiful, but it was just so hard to keep the instrument from clenching up, and I was feeling things, and I was just. . . . *(sigh)*

Int: Did you feel comfortable telling your teacher that?

JT: Um, I think so, maybe not in so many words but I think so. We had a conversation about it, because we were searching for something that would feel good, I guess. So I think I remember articulating that whatever it was, it wasn't pants roles.

Int: Right! Whatever it is, it's not this.

JT: Or like, I was trying but I couldn't. I think we talked about it. It's interesting because it's very clearly a woman's role, even if that role is playing a boy or something, it's not written for a male, and it's not supposed to actually be perceived as a male. From an identity perspective, that's what a trans person adamantly *is not* is a woman in men's clothes, you know?

Int: Exactly. Have there been other times when you've felt like others saw you that way, artistically or even in your fellow musician communities at work?

JT: Probably. There are times I feel that way just in life in general. Now it's less that way. Most of my colleagues now, and in graduate school after I came out, have been great. It's more stressful around people that know me less well or don't have to work with me every day or are just less well educated on it. For the most part, the new music scene is pretty well educated on social issues. There are blind spots for sure, and it varies from person to person, but nobody wants to be that person that doesn't understand trans issues. You know, when, in our field, there's a fight for relevance all the time.

Int: Of course. Do you ever feel like your family sees you still as a woman in men's clothing?

JT: Yeah. I have family members who see me that way, you know? Even if it's not perceptible that someone is seeing me that way, that's the fear I guess, because that is what people think of trans people when they don't understand, you know? That we're imposters, or mentally unstable.

Int: How do you think your voice impacts that perception with your family?

JT: Maybe. It's hard to tell if it's my voice specifically, because they're evolving on their own too, you know, and I look different, and there's a lot of factors. There have been times, like visits home, where I've found it easier or harder for whatever reason to speak comfortably in a lower register. But I think it does affect both how comfortable I am, and how they seem to be receiving me when I do it successfully.

Int: What are some other times when it's easier to let your voice sit a little bit lower and times when it's harder to let that happen? Can you talk a little about that, maybe specifically when you're teaching?

JT: Sure, yeah. I think I'm kind of in the middle of it now, of finding a way to present myself in a teaching situation that conveys caring for my students without defaulting to female modes of speech to express that.

Int: Have you found anything that's worked yet?

JT: It's getting easier, I think. There's one colleague who has a really clear, low, booming voice and also comes across as a nice person. He's one who I've found myself studying the way he talks a little bit.

Int: Do you do that with singers too? Make models of singers that you like?

JT: A little bit. Maybe pop singers, Sam Smith probably, although now, that's starting to be too high, but yeah, just the way that he sings. I don't know, there are other cases where I'm singing along with someone who I wouldn't necessarily want to sound like, but I'm still noticing what it is about their production that's different than mine. When I was singing Tamino I was listening to classical tenors a little.

Int: Do you have visions for your voice? Do you know what you would want it to sound like? Or what you hope it will sound like?

JT: I'm not sure I do 100% yet, but maybe. I think it's getting a little clearer as it seems more possible, but I'm still figuring that out. I think a pleasant, clear, slightly gay-sounding baritone speaking voice is probably what I would like.

Int: And how do you define that?

JT: Yeah I don't know . . . I think of a couple people actually who speak that way, not like famous people but, um I don't know. The gay-sounding part would be the part that I'd have to define for myself, right? Like pleasant, and clear, and baritone—but I think there're a number of things that could be heard as "gay-sounding," and they're not all things that I would want in the way that I speak, so I guess yeah, I should clarify. It's not like a register and it's not like a nasal edge, it's more just an inflection I guess. I'm not worried about the fact my [s] sounds or [t] sounds come across as feminine. I do sort of speak a little bit tersely and pretty directly, and that's probably a family thing. All that will probably still be there, but I'm also drawn to people who speak a little bit more slowly and with more contour, and draw out their vowels a little more and that goes along with a pleasant, clear quality for me.

Int: And then do you have the same kind of vision for your singing voice? Or do you know yet?

JT: I don't know yet, I don't think, maybe some similar things. I don't want it especially affected toward any one genre. I want it very versatile and clarity is an important quality for me. I don't know if I'm going to end up a tenor or a baritone or what, right?

Int: You'll end up as you! And wherever your voice evolves next, you've said that you still want to explore your higher range and all the parts up there. Have you ever felt like you wanted to abandon or remove that part of your voice?

JT: That's an interesting question. I don't think so. The uppermost part of it I actually am probably more comfortable with than the lyric soprano C4–G5 register. When I'm in the uppermost parts, especially above high B, it almost gets to a point where it's superhuman more than female, I guess. Especially now I think it's kind of cool that my voice is producing those harmonics.

Int: And those uppermost notes are happening spontaneously now, right?

JT: Yeah! My range is growing on both ends, it's just kind of turning into [crap] in the middle. *(Laughter)* But I don't mind the top part, and as I'm practicing I'm usually more reluctant to work with A4–G5 than to see what might come out above that.

Int: Is that reluctance about feeling unsteady, or about not liking the way it sounds, or are those related?

JT: Maybe both. It used to be not liking the way it sounded or the way that it felt for me to sound that way. Now it also just is physically uncomfortable and strange sounding. I'm probably less worried about the gender implications now that I feel a little bit more secure that I'm going to be able to leave all that behind or am in the process of doing that. Ideally, I'd like to keep all that range. It'd be really amazing if it happened that way, to come out of this with a five-octave range.

Int: Your current hormone dose is very low, and you are taking your time with this part of transition. How does that feel? You've mentioned feeling simultaneously impatient while also acknowledging that it's the right choice to go slow.

JT: Yeah I'm in the middle of that. It very much depends on how things are going that day. I don't know, a week ago I was like, "I can take my time, the voice is the most important thing," and right after a voice lesson that's probably how I feel. Right after getting misgendered repeatedly, though, I am beginning to get impatient with it. I just moved; I don't necessarily have a close relationship with a doctor yet and it's hard to know what I should be doing.

Int: What of the resources that you have read through and consumed about hormonal transition and voice has been helpful? What information do you look for?

JT: I'm trying to look for what dosage people were on at what point, and how well they felt like things were going for their voice, and I know it's different for everybody so it's hard to know what to do with that information but it's been somewhat useful.

Int: While living in Chicago, you were able to come sing with Resonate for a little while, but now since there is not a trans choir in your area, do you have a community of music folks who have similar experiences to you? Is having a group like a trans choir something that you would want or need in your life?

JT: That's a good question. There's probably very few people in the world who are not only going through this but are professional musicians as well, you know? It can sometimes be hard to have something that I do for fun that is similar to what I do in work, but at a slower pace that aligns with everyone else in the group.

Int: Do you then have to choose between feeding your singer identity and feeding a desire to have a community of gender-diverse folks around you? And would singing in an all-trans choir feel like reducing your singing voice to your gender identity? Did you ever feel that way in Resonate?

JT: What was weird about it at that time, before I started T, was that I was one of two soprano voices. It was definitely me and the one other high voice sticking out over this whole other lower part, and it did feel a little awkward. But I think that the other high voice singer came to love it, and I didn't necessarily not enjoy it, but it was weird. I would like to know more trans singers, but I know a lot of singers who are sympathetic to this and curious about it, and then I also know a lot of LGBT people so, I guess I have a community there.

Int: If doing online lessons wasn't possible, how would you have gone about finding a teacher in your new town?

JT: I don't know!

Int: What would you look for in a new teacher now?

JT: I guess there were a number of factors but it became clear the most important one was cultural competence in this area. I don't know what I'd be doing if I hadn't found a teacher, but I'd probably be informally singing with people. I figured I'd come here and just try to find the queer community in general and hopefully there would be singers or, if nothing else, strong allies.

Int: In thinking about a scenario in which you would have to educate your educator on cultural competence, how do you feel about that?

JT: I don't know. I mean, I guess I was thinking of it more from a technical standpoint in terms of my voice changes. I teach all the time, so when I think about that I guess I'm thinking more about explaining what might be happening technically and less about a scenario where I'm explaining how I might be feeling. I imagine that would just come up in the moment. I didn't have to teach my current voice teacher about that, it was always just a priority and I actually think I learned that the emotional side is important through that experience.

Int: What did you feel like you could talk through in lessons that you didn't expect to?

JT: Your instrument is your body when you're a singer, so how you're feeling on a certain day and how everything else is going in your life affects how you come into a voice lesson. I think a major strength of my teacher for me, and I'm sure other trans singers, is that we always make it a point to pick up on the life stuff and not just focus on the vocal aspect. It's very important, especially when one's comfort in a specific register is tied to how they feel about themselves in that moment, in the repertoire they're singing and in how their life is going. It's actually is directly related, you know?

Int: When you talk about cultural competency, what does that look like to you? How would you know that you were in a situation with a culturally competent teacher?

JT: I would prefer not to explain the big important, obvious things like: I am actually a man, I'm not just someone who wants to be one, and what vocal dysphoria even is or might be. It's very intangible, but I think a lot of teachers who might be working with a trans student for the first time are capable of that kind of understanding, so it's not something you would necessarily find on a résumé. I've also met people whose job it is to work with trans people show a shocking level of cultural incompetence, so it just kind of depends I guess. I was talking to a voice teacher at the faculty cookout a few weeks into the new year, and she told me she had been working with a trans student and it was her first time working with anybody who's not cis. She didn't know the right pronouns, and she was struggling to talk about this person, but I could tell that she was a good teacher for them. She said, "You know I think you just are what you are, your voice is really unique, but more importantly, we should follow your heart and work with you where you are." I think she's a really good teacher for this student.

Int: Sure, like somebody who at least has a compassionate way of moving through the world—

JT: Yeah, just an open perspective.

Int: Going back to the idea of explaining technically what's going on with your voice as you go through hormonal transition, what would it be like to have a teacher who was less knowledgeable about the anatomy, physiology, and function of your voice, specifically, as a trans man on T?

JT: It would be hard. I'd be reading a lot as I am, but that'd be hard. That's sort of what I was looking for, what I was hoping to find more than anything. I guess I tend to feel like I can take care of the emotional side, whether or not that's true, but I just want someone that knows what the [heck] is going on. I have a friend who teaches voice and among her students are adolescent boys. I was talking to her a bit about this, just describing what I thought was happening, and she's like, "Yeah it just sounds like an adolescent boy" and I knew it was different but I didn't know how to explain that it's different. So that could be challenging if a teacher were to say something like that to me. Because then I wouldn't know if I could trust their instinct on what we were doing or if they would have an understanding of how to offer information about dosages, that aspect I'd be on my own with.

Int: That sounds really scary. If a teacher said, "Oh it's just this. Simple."

JT: Right, "it's just like this" and you kind of have a sense that it's not, but part of me is wondering if it is.

Int: Flipping that around, as an educator who works in academia, do you see instances of cultural competency in your colleagues? Do you wish that there was a different level of cultural competency in your colleagues, specifically in the music department?

JT: I think they're pretty great. It's funny because it varies. The school as a whole is trying really hard right now to be culturally competent in every aspect of identity politics. I went through LGBT Safe Zone training so that I could put a plaque on my office door that says it's an LGBT safe zone and that people can come talk to me. It's kind of hilarious because I feel like I'm a walking LGBT safe zone. I mean, it could've been worse but the training definitely could've been a lot better.

The discussion of gender was just like, "Look at this picture of a Barbie and this picture of an action figure and discuss."

Int: No way.

JT: "And here's a bunch of terms, bathrooms are important, and trans students don't feel safe, we need to help them feel safe" but that was pretty much it. There was more on gay and lesbian issues and they were like a *little* better about that. So I have my plaque now, and the head of the music department is encouraging all of us to have them because it's really important to him that LGBT students feel like the music department is a safe place for them. My colleagues have been awesome and made several of the bathrooms gender neutral.

Int: Are there policies for students, for example, for preferred name, pronouns, and contact information?

JT: They do have that, which is nice. I'm seeing that as an evolution. My graduate school had that to some degree, but if I hadn't legally changed my name and continued to teach there I would've shown up as [*given name*] in their course system.

Int: But they couldn't just change it for you because you asked them to?

JT: They could change it on some things, but not everything for some reason. It seemed to be an IT issue, or nobody knew how, or they just don't do that until you make a legal name change, then somehow, they find a way to make the effort.

Int: That's unacceptable.

JT: Yeah.

Int: Do you know what the student policies are like at your new university yet?

JT: Students can designate their preferred name and preferred pronouns and they'll only show up in any of the systems as that name. They did a better job with that. In terms of individual colleagues, for the most part, I've been misgendered a couple of times and everybody's really apologetic if they do it. For the most part I feel that everybody's hearts are in the right place and some of them actually are allies in the queer community and really understand. I feel lucky, it's a younger and cooler faculty than I might've found myself working with in a lot of places.

Int: What would you say to teachers and students, what would you want them to know?

JT: Maybe it's a little easier for teachers, they should try their best to have as deep of an understanding of trans people as possible and also to think about their own gender identity and gender presentation. The problem is when somebody sees the trans person as abnormal, rather than just on a spectrum that we're all on somewhere, navigating how we present ourselves to the world and think about ourselves. I think I'm the least comfortable in a situation if someone is trying to be very nice and accommodating but also clearly sees me as a special case in need of accommodation. For students, I might be able to answer that better once I'm on the other side of most of the changing that's happening with my voice. I know I was really afraid to start testosterone, but now I'm really happy that I'm on this path. I'm also happy that I waited until I was sure I really wanted to do it. I spent 2 years figuring out more about my relationship to my voice, and attempting to physically transition as much as I could on my own so that now it's less of an uphill battle. I'm happy that I listened to myself at every stage and tried to figure out what it was that I really needed. When you come out as trans, there's a lot of noise from everywhere, even from the community, about how you should be doing it and what you need to do. Transition really is very individual and different for everybody so don't necessarily listen to anyone; learn what you need to learn and figure it out.

Int: At what point did you go from not having language to talk about how you were feeling to having that language and knowledge, where did that happen for you?

JT: I've been writing in journals since I was 10, maybe that's something that I'm somewhat good at, therapy is awesome, everybody should go to therapy if they can. It definitely is helpful to bring people in. Taking voice lessons has been important for me because I wasn't going to be able to have a clear perspective on my own of how I felt about my voice and what I wanted my voice to be. The more you can bring in knowledgeable, supportive people, the better.

Int: Anything else that you want to share, or say?

JT: I can't think of anything.

Int: Okay. Thank you, JT.

JT: You're welcome. Thank YOU.

ALEXA GRÆ

ALEXA holds a master's degree in voice performance from Northwestern University and is an active professional singer, songwriter, performer, and voice teacher. ALEXA began working with transgender and nonbinary singers and speakers in the spring of 2017 and has a full schedule of predominantly gender-diverse students. ALEXA is uniquely adept at holding space for their students to explore identity and voice, while allowing room to process new pedagogical challenges as a teacher. After this interview, ALEXA discussed the revelation of finally being able to link some of the uncomfortable experiences throughout the early part of their singing career to some dysphoria about their own voice.

Int: indicates the interviewers

ALEXA: indicates the student's response

Int: Can you talk a little bit about your singing life?

ALEXA: I've been signing since I was a child. I really got into singing when I was 6 or 7 years old, in church. It was just me and Mom growing up, and she was in the church choir. I got really bored sitting in the pew by myself while she was singing, and I could carry a tune, so I got to sing with my mom for a really long time. I started doing solos, and then I started taking piano lessons. I was in choirs my whole life, then went to study in college and thought I'd like to be a famous musician, like an R&B singer. My freshman year in college was the first time I ever saw an opera. It was the most human, and sometimes inhuman, or otherworldly, connection to human drama. So, I went from only singing classically in choirs to then singing R&B and pop, and then eventually started bringing both worlds together.

Int: You do so much varied musical work, can you talk a little bit about your own creative style?

ALEXA: Sure. I think my creative style pulls from different worlds. I think there are pieces of R&B, some jazziness, in a very classical idiom. In undergrad, I was a composition major and I started writing classical instrumental pieces, and then finally started writing for choir and voice. The first piece I ever wrote for myself was a super art song on steroids. It's very French, mysterious, dark, and it really was the first time I could point to the way I wanted to sing, the way I want to present this voice, this instrument, this body. And that's sort of why I started writing for myself, because at the time, I wasn't connecting to the literature or characters that were specifically written for my voice type.

Int: What has been your journey with your voice type?

ALEXA: My voice changed a lot in high school. I entered high school still being able to sing soprano, but I didn't want anyone to yell at me, so I sang tenor. Then I went to undergrad as a tenor. Eventually, I had a conversation with my teacher and said that I would love to sing something a little higher, so I brought in some Purcell. But even then, I still was like, "mmm it's not high enough," and my teacher brought in the *Chichester Psalms* by Bernstein, the second movement boy soprano solo, and I started singing and we were both like, "yes!"

Int: Nice!

ALEXA: Yeah, and it started this interesting road. My teacher showed me all the standard counter tenor rep and I was into some of it, but most of the early music I didn't really care for. The stuff I remember bringing to him freshmen year was Strauss and Rachmaninoff, and all this romantic, wading in the emotional waters stuff, and he was like, "uuuh, I don't think ya know who ya are."

Int: Did you feel like you knew who you were?

ALEXA: Yeah. I think I did, I just think that where I was singing as an 18-year-old, my voice wasn't going to do that yet. But my teachers basically told me that early music was all there was. I could see that from a teaching standpoint, but they might not have known what else was out there, you know? I'm not upset about it now. I went into that realm halfheartedly.

Int: The counter tenor realm?

ALEXA: Yeah because at least it felt really good to sing there. I wasn't crazy about all the rep, so there was a lot of push and pull with my teacher. He let me sing some rep that I enjoyed, but he would also say, "You have to sing this, too."

Int: Do you do think that he didn't want to give you too much heavy repertoire at a young age as a measure of vocal health, or do you think he was trying to box you into a Fach?

ALEXA: I think it was a choice for vocal health. I also think it was maybe to coax me into it, he thought I might like it if I just gave it a chance. So, I left my undergrad working on early music and really trying to find art song, because I was crazy about art song. I was trying to find means to express myself in a different way, that I personally wasn't discovering in the realm of early music. Regardless of his intention, I felt boxed.

Int: Did the same feeling come up in your choral ensembles? What part did you sing when you were in choir?

ALEXA: I sang Alto II. I'm not an Alto II; kind of an alto, but kind of a soprano. I need some lightness or my voice gets really tired in that register.

Int: So even in undergrad, it sounds like the idea of the "boy soprano" didn't fit, and that may have been linked to gender expression in voice. When do you think that process started for you?

ALEXA: Hmm. I feel like it was probably there, early on, but I don't think I had the language to really talk about what was going on subconsciously. There's something about singing high and how my body responds—it feels so free. I have a flexibility there that feels like I couldn't really get anywhere else in my range. I don't think until maybe grad school was the term "falsetto" used to describe my voice. I don't really like that term. As I was getting older, every time it was used I was like, "yuck." Like I could feel my body react to that word. Because it doesn't feel fake or false, it feels like a part of my voice I have access to, and it feels like my expressions are maximized here. So, I sort of checked in with that feeling. I think it really started happening as I got closer to graduation, figuring out what I was auditioning for, and there were opera programs, but I wasn't seeing anything that would fit. I was realizing my voice does not sit in normal counter tenor land, wondering if these programs I was thinking about would cast a male-bodied individual to play a pants role. Not seeing any outlets, I didn't see where I would fit in. Then I started writing for myself like, "Well if nobody's gonna write it for you, you gotta do it yourself."

Int: And it sounds like even the repertoire that might have fit with your voice technically at the time was not in line with the characters you wanted to play. Can you talk a little about the types of characters you're drawn to?

ALEXA: I think I was more interested in playing myself or playing pieces of me than a character, especially a character with old narratives. I'm a lover or a romantic and I wanted to at least be that person. A lot of the roles that were designed for my voice type didn't match my temperament. When I was singing tenor, I did a lot of comedic roles and it was fun, but then as I was getting older I wanted something a little more serious. When I'm writing for myself, I use words that my mom wrote and that's where my concept of femme psyche comes from, and it feels really good in my voice. That has made a big difference for me in terms of connecting to a character, or developing a relationship with a character. Another theme that sometimes shows up for me is something like a soliloquy, from roles like Orfeo or Oberon where the character kind of comes in and does their thing and then leaves. Now, in my own art song, I'm singing *to* something but not really about anyone or with anyone. I don't necessarily know who I want to sing to, I just want it to be an experience for everyone.

Int: Can you say a little more about femme psyche? How do you think that has shown up in your art?

ALEXA: Femme for me is strength in vulnerability. I think of the great divas, and we love them for walking up to the edge and staying there for hours at a time. There's something about that power that I find so interesting and inspiring—diving into your art, diving into your voice, diving into your own sound and gifting it to other people, or creating a world that they can come into.

Int: And it sounds like your mom gave you an avenue into that. Can you say a little more about your mom and how she influences your music?

ALEXA: So, the first piece I wrote for voice was a choral piece and I remember talking to my mom, asking for advice or favorite poems and she was like, "Oh well I've written some" and pulls out 30-something poems! I went to read through them and thought, "This is it." It's so intense and it's from a dark time in my mom's life, a romantic time, like a breakup. And she was brave enough to even share this with her child, which, I felt like was a lot already. I decided to have it translated into French, because that gives a little bit of a barrier for my mom's vulnerable words to her child, respecting the words, and giving myself some space to say them truthfully. I asked my aunt to translate it. I love the French language. I love the way it feels in my mouth, in my body. And at a time when I was starting to really claim my authentic voice, whatever that means, I needed that little bit of a veil, of not singing it in English, to be able to express the words in this very real way, kind of for the first time.

Int: Do you think that poetry helped you identify and connect with your own femme psyche?

ALEXA: Absolutely, yeah. I think it was really like, the character that emerged was my mom and me, that's who that is. It's not Cherubino, it's not Oberon the King, it's a melding of worlds and this connection between child and mother telling a story.

Int: How do you think that melding of worlds shows up in other ways?

ALEXA: As a performer, I started with my best friends from grad school and we formed a group, delving into worlds that we felt like we didn't get to play in during grad school like queer identity, sex positivity, things that make up our culture outside of school and rep, combined with heightened artistic training. When I was with them my name was GRÆ at the time, which actually came from notes I started writing on social media 10 years earlier about "the space in between," about my background of being African-American-Caucasian, and also what music looks like in those two worlds between "high art" and "pop." And then after a year, after I had that name, I knew it felt like a placeholder, it didn't feel quite right. My roommates were always calling me Alexa or Lexi. So, ALEXA GRÆ emerged, and it sounds like a superhero.

Int: How do you manage stepping into and out of that femme psyche on a day-to-day basis? How do you express it? How do people react to it?

ALEXA: I think it's really getting more comfortable with myself. Sort of like being unbothered. And also, when you seem confident, when you can tell that other people see it, they pick up on that energy. But I think my in-between-ness is what I gravitate towards. There's something about it that just is, just the shape. It's not a gender, it's a shape. If I could just be a shape, I'd be a shape. I'd be many shapes, versus feeling like I'm putting on this shirt and it feels gendered. It's a structure to cover my body. I've always dressed the way I wanted to. . . . Actually, not always. A few years ago, a lot changed in my world and I started questioning my own gender. I had a lot of loss that year, but that summer I had really found my tribe and friends, my queers. I felt really safe for the first time. And my style changed, it was more flowy and more femme, it was more like *Neverland* Peter Pan. That same year, my grandmother passed away, and I was going back to South Texas. It was my first time stepping back into that church again after years. I remember my mom was kind of like, "Of course you're gonna wear a tie and suit" and I hated it. I wanted to rip that stuff off my skin. Going down there, putting on a sports coat and a tie and just—I hated it. I hated it. I didn't want to put it on, but I also did *not* want to be stared at so I just did it. And I didn't want to answer questions like, "Why are you dressed like that? Why are your nails painted?" My grandmother died, I wasn't in the mood to discuss my appearance. It was so many things. My grandmother was Southern Baptist and there were a lot of things she didn't get. Whatever. Love her. Even if she didn't understand it, she always wanted me to be me. My mom too, from a very young age, was like "just be you." And I also realize that growing up, when I was taking music lessons, I mean I was playing the piano at 10:45 in the evening, and she'd be in the next room watching *Golden Girls* or something and say, "That's pretty!" and I was, you know, banging on the piano and singing as loud as I could. My mom never told me to shut up. She never told me to be quiet. A lot of that didn't happen until I was in school, or even at gigs, where people would pick apart my voice and ask for certain sounds—and the sounds they wanted were small and only fit a narrow scope of what I could do. I kept hearing "tone that down" or "you have to sing this way" or "don't use that voice, it sounds like a woman," so I'm kind of uncovering that. I'd say I was insanely blessed and gifted for my mom and my grandmother. The women in my family are incredibly inspiring. . . . Anyway. I think when we put on clothes, it's our armor to go face the world. I remember doing a performance and really diving into the Diva in this hyper-femme sort of state, and then being done with that project and then my whole wardrobe changed. I felt like I needed to be hidden from the world. When I dove into the Diva, I was really aware of the way the world *sees* you constantly, and I felt more seen as femme; people talking to me, warm smiles, but at the same time quick to criticize or comment on how I looked or acted—and then being able to be invisible or anonymous was something I did through my clothes. My clothes were reflecting how I was feeling that day. Right now, I feel like I'm leaning more towards a neutral, body-agnostic wardrobe. This feels like my normal state, that's what those shapes feel like. It's this neutral gray sort of thing.

Int: What about in your voice? How do you express your gender with your voice?

ALEXA: I think my speaking voice is up and down a lot. I feel kind of child-like in range and pitch, and that matches my singing. I sing in my upper registers and I also try to use all of my voice all the time. It's not just one thing, it's all of me.

Int: Have you ever felt dysphoric about your voice?

ALEXA: A few times. I don't think I actually had the language back then. I have had a few times where I've been singing something, not sure if it's real—not so much out-of-body or anything, but "false." Sometimes I would sing and wonder if it was me, or if I was creating something that wasn't truth, that wasn't grounded, that felt like a trick or gag. I think there were a few times like that in school. But I put on a good face for a very long time. Even though I thought I knew better than my teachers about what my voice does, I would go home and have no idea what was going on. When there were no outlets, no real places where I would use this type of singing, I wondered what I was even doing making those sounds. I feel like that's my dysphoria. Once I leaned into loving all of my voice, it went away and I embraced everything my voice could do.

Int: When are the times when you feel the least safe singing?

ALEXA: Once, I elected to say yes to an audition for a local opera company in Chicago. I hadn't done an opera in forever, and the audition presented itself. I used this experience to try it and see how I liked it; I wasn't getting any other work and it fit my voice range. I can say, on the other side of it, I'm glad I did it to learn about myself but it was the most unsafe I've ever felt and it had nothing to do with anybody in the production. It was all internal. I was so focused on making perfect sound that I was caged in my own voice, and all the things that I teach to my own students about getting out of their own way, I just could not. Things that I had done to unlock my voice were not working. I was so stressed for a good 2 months straight and I kept thinking, "I have to make it through this, I never want to feel like this again." Even the range wasn't good. I'd practice and practice, but it wasn't showing up, it wasn't in my voice. There was no way around it. I remember the very first night, and almost crying as soon as I stepped onstage. All of a sudden, I couldn't even remember the Italian. The first line started and a tear was about to fall out of my eye. The music came, but I never felt safe during the entire performance. We had four shows in a row and I didn't think of what that would do to me and every night got harder and harder. I was embarrassed. It was the first time I'd ever felt embarrassed about a performance. My family all came in and they thought it was great, and to be honest I don't think it sounded as bad as it was in my head, but knowing that I couldn't enjoy myself onstage was the biggest red flag. A few months later, I got asked to do a gig singing Spanish early music. I'd done it before and recorded it and thought it would be fine. And I needed the money. In the days leading up to the performance, I was nauseous and I could tell something was happening emotionally. I had to sing this rep that wasn't for my voice and it did not sit well. At the concert, I was up there singing a few solos but having a reaction like, "Oh god this is just like the opera. You're feeling the same way but you're looking at a score." It was terrible. I remember coughing in the middle of a run and I wasn't even choking, I didn't know what was going on. I was putting myself through torture. I think that was the second scare, enough to say, "No more. Stop doing things that you're told you're supposed to sing because they fit your voice, because they don't. They don't fit, and until you're good with that, don't do it. You're not far enough away from it. Not moved passed it enough." I learned those feelings are bigger than just performing. I haven't done anything like that since then, and I started to really focus on my own stuff after that.

Int: What do you tend to write about in your own music?

ALEXA: I ask a lot of questions in my music and my lyrics. I think it's from doing work on gender identity and stuff with myself, and asking questions so I know where I'm at right now. The questions are like, "I if I share something, can you take care of this? Will you hold it and keep it sacred, or will you hurt me? I'm presenting to you who I am, what are you going to do with it?" In the grand scheme of academia, and lovers, family, friends, that's what I feel like a lot of the music is about. I feel like it's a mix. One line can be from one story, the next line will be from a completely different story and it goes back and forth. It's a lot of questions.

Int: What do you hope the answers will be?

ALEXA: That's a good question. I think I definitely remember a turning point in the music that I created with a song called "The Prince." In the first half I had fallen, feeling some kind of way about a close friend and they were gone for the summer, and I was asking, "Where is my prince, who created this beautiful world for us to exist in?" And there was a falling out and then I looked at the song again and I realized I was the one who created this universe. I created the happiness. I think

I still ask questions but that's for the listener to answer. It's interesting to see what you'll say, but I've got to do my thing. There's a line that I use from James Agee's "Knoxville Summer of 1915" from a child's perspective: "After a little I am taken in and put to bed, sleep soft, smiling draws me under her and those who quietly treat me as one familiar and well-beloved in that home, but will not, not now, not ever, tell me who I am." I've heard enough from everybody's input, of my voice, of my gender.

Int: That's a good segue into your teaching life because there's a shared experience among us, as teachers, where we are witness to and part of the same process with our students as singers and as people, specifically as gender-diverse people. What are some moments when you've seen your own experience mirrored in your students?

ALEXA: I had a student, and I could see they were getting frustrated and couldn't get out of their own way. And then all of a sudden, I was thinking about that experience in the opera. I couldn't ask this student the same thing my director asked of me. I wasn't going to ask my student to perform, I wanted them to be themselves. I felt like I had to explain some things and say, "I want you to know that this will always be open and when you're ready, I'm going to try to invite you, but I'm not going to push you." There's so much more going on than just a sound, so I want to create the most welcoming and inviting space. Also, I know I'm going to mess up and find places where my own issues come up that I have to work through and not push that on anybody else. Identity is wrapped up in this instrument and there's not a one-size-fits-all. There are so many different facets and things that inform the way we sing that are greater than any one voice lesson.

Int: What do you think have been some of the differences in working with trans and nonbinary singers compared to your teaching life before?

ALEXA: In grad school, I was teaching a bunch of music theater kids who were in performance mode all the time and sometimes had to learn pieces quickly before a show. There was as much vocal health as I could throw in, of course. For those students, there was always a need to perform, always putting on a mask, and there was so little time for honesty in those lessons. I think now, having so many students here for discovery, they're here to look into the darkness and find who they are, unlock things, and that's different. It's more about getting to the core. They're not hiding behind characterizations, they're coming here with pieces that are missing. It's a different kind of patience, it really is. This is long game. I've been wondering why I was so guarded with my previous voice teachers and didn't have the language and didn't feel safe—I loved both of them, but I never had a moment of breaking down and being really vulnerable. I never experienced that. And I hear so much of it now from my own students. I want them to be honest and truthful, and having students come in and have little breakdowns, that's expected now. I'm glad that I get to see that and partake, or be there with that person.

Int: Do you ever find this work overwhelming?

ALEXA: The first two times I cried after teaching lessons it was from witnessing sheer bravery. Having people go to explore, to look into the darkness, find something they want to improve upon, find an outlet, and find something to connect even more with themselves and their identity is so brave. And I know I had a different kind of outlet that was masked and guarded but was able to work itself out—not in a room with one person, but in performance sometimes or in queer, hippie spaces. It was very different. So, for my students to come in here week after week and sit by the piano with me is incredible. Mostly I cry from joy, but there have been a few times that I was overwhelmed by somebody's situation, like, how are they functioning, and realizing how much energy I have to have to support that. Every day is a little different. Teaching is so important for me, and I want to help people. And on the other side, I'm such a performer and creator I feel like I'm at my best when I'm also teaching my students how to do it.

Int: Going back to the idea of voice types, have you ever had a student who wanted to sing in a range that you thought would be unhealthy?

ALEXA: Yes.

Int: How did you navigate that?

ALEXA: I have had students or other individuals who don't identify as trans or [gender nonconforming] who tell me where they want to sing and I'm always asking why. It's not for me to decide, we work together on it. I think you can teach it in a manner that gives students both freedom and vocal health, and it's really up to them to decide if they want to stay there, or try a different place in their voice, or use all of it. For me, a lot of teaching is trying to give all the crayons and let the students make their own picture.

Int: How might you work with someone who has limited access to the range that they want to be singing in, but has severe dysphoria about singing in a range that might be healthier?

ALEXA: I would be checking in constantly. I'm not going to try to lead them to where they don't want to be for a while. I definitely need to build trust so they'll let me help them get there. I would ask questions like, "What would it feel like to sit in this dysphoria for a little bit?" And then be incredibly transparent, letting them know "this is what I hear, can you tell me how it feels?" I want to at least mirror or reflect some of what I think is going on.

Int: Have you ever had that experience for yourself as a student, that someone would walk you through different parts of your range and ask how it felt?

ALEXA: Uh-uh no. I didn't really even talk about my own emotions or any thoughts that I had. I might have said, "I think this poem is pretty" or say something about a piece, but for the most part I wasn't sharing.

Int: Do you think that was related to the way you had been moving through the world? There's the stereotypical notion that women are more emotional than men; do you think that was related?

ALEXA: I think it actually feels more race related. Being a person of color, I was always trying not to make excuses, trying not to look weak. I *hate* that word, and that notion of having to present in a masculine way. Also, being a person of color or black biracial, I always thought I had to be better at so many other things, better than other people, or be seen as constant and steady rather than emotional.

Int: If you met a teacher who said they were really interested in what you do, and would like to start working with trans/gnc singers, what would you tell them?

ALEXA: I don't know if I would tell them anything, but I think I would ask questions. I would ask, "Why, what is your reason?" Because I feel like if the answer is, "Oh that sounds cool," then it's a little iffy.

Int: The word "fascinating" in reference to trans people is turning into sort of a trigger word.

ALEXA: Yeah! And I can get that from a pedagogical place, but also, they're human, we're all human, talk to us like humans.

Maybe start there, and soul search. Soul. Search. It's more commitment than you could imagine. It's a lot of brain space that gets taken up and there's a lot of heart space that gets taken up.

Int: If you were going to talk to singing students, what would you say to them? To the up-and-coming trans and nonbinary singers?

ALEXA: Your path is your own. You've *got* to make your own and I know it's hard without other paths to see, but look further, someone has a lantern on, somebody's holding a light, just keep going. The hardest road to forge is your own, but know that, and it becomes a thing that you do and you stay on your path.

Int: Thank you so much, ALEXA.

ALEXA: Yeah, my pleasure.

REGINA

Regina has been a singer her entire life. Recently retired, she spends her weekday evenings singing in a local chorus and at karaoke nights at local bars with friends. She is bigender and lives her life as both a man and a woman in different situations. She sings as her male self in the choral group, and she takes voice lessons as her female self. She says there are different voices, different ways of learning, and different ways of moving through the world between her male and female selves. Often, discovering her best techniques as a singer involves acknowledging the different ways she learned to sing as a tenor and reapplying that information to her new repertoire as a mezzo-soprano.

One of the most interesting insights Regina has had about her voice education is that sometimes when she's in lessons as her female self, aspects of her male self and the way he maneuvers vulnerable situations affect her ability to take on new skills. As a Black man growing up in the projects of Chicago, he developed physically and emotionally protective mechanisms to keep himself safe and alive during the most trying parts of his life. Now, whenever there are new challenges—even in a place as seemingly innocuous as voice lessons—if there is a sense that there may be danger, or vulnerability, or lack of control, the masculine parts of Regina's identity come forward. Her mannerisms and physicality change, her tone of voice changes, or she pauses sometimes to process what is being asked of her while she sings. It takes a moment and she doesn't always notice it at first, but she can recognize that shift and bring herself back to full presence and mindfulness.

The voice studio is an inherently vulnerable space, and she is learning how to inhabit that vulnerable space fully as herself. She has a bubbly, loquacious personality and the joy that comes from singing is genuine and bright. Developing new exercises that are more like songs than vocalises and choosing repertoire that aligns completely with her sense of self are helping her define successful voice education on her own terms. In this interview, she talks about navigating her own expectations about her voice and the myriad challenges she faces as a bigender singer living in two separate worlds.

Int: indicates the interviewers

Regina: indicates the student's response

Int: Can you talk a little bit about your singing life?

Regina: I love to sing, I LOVE to sing! It's my favorite thing to do. If I couldn't sing I don't know what I would do, I can't imagine. I want to sing better always, on the one hand. But truly, people love to hear me sing. They think I'm talented. They do.

Int: You are!

Glory *(Flattered laughter)* But I always hear all the things that are wrong and I always want to do better. I would say I love the fact that my voice has a lot of range. I can sing songs that are fairly low, and songs that are pretty high. But there are parts of my voice that I don't like, and I have become aware of the limitations and the things that I can do to make it better, but it's work.

Int: You have been singing your whole life, and you are a performer and your performance life is varied. You have the choir, and you do karaoke among other things . . .

Regina: And the majority of the time I sing as a male, but at times I also sing as a female. I want to be authentic each way which is difficult, and I think I ask a lot of myself in that. But yes, I sing in every opportunity that's presented to me.

Int: How do you think voice lessons are impacting your performance life? What are some ways that different techniques are showing up for you?

Regina: I think the things that I've learned work in a funda-mental way so that no matter what I'm doing, it helps. I'm in a chorus and we had a show recently, and I was just getting over a cold and I had to sing really high in my chest voice. It really was a struggle for me but the way that I worked through it was through breath support and actually, I cheated a little as I was singing. When I was coming to the part when I had to go high, I took a quick breath so I could maintain the note better. And when I do karaoke, for example, there are songs I wouldn't have sung before, but breath support helps me do that. As a woman singing, it's still a work in progress but I try to add more color to my female voice as I sing. That's harder for me because it's so much a departure from what I've done in the past. But those are the ways, I think, the big things that have been helpful to me.

Int: In discovering a feminine singing voice you've been learning how to sing with different colors, even in the parts of your range that overlap with your tenor voice. What do you think are some of the things that allow you to do that, to use different vocal colors in the same pitch range?

Regina: The technical parts are bringing the sound from a dif-ferent place so it doesn't sound so thin, and having it higher in my head but also trying to have it more rounded in my head or my mouth. When it's more rounded it sounds fuller and it sounds totally different when I do that. It's still work for me. I think I'm still early with that. Before I started lessons, I wasn't ever aware of that at all, so for example, I would sing songs as a woman and I could sing them in the right key, but I had no idea that I could change the color of it, make it fuller. So at least I'm aware and I can do that, but it's harder because the sound is so new to me. I have to work through that. Some-times, it sounds artificial to me and it could be because it's too new or because I'm doing too much of it.

Int: Can you say more about that? There's a little bit of identity wrapped up in that, it seems. Can you talk a little bit about some of the things you're exploring with how different it is to sing as your female self?

Regina: Well, we were talking about the technical aspects, but then there's the psychological part. I'm always aware that I have to pull Regina's voice more to the front, and that makes all of this easier. You know, the struggle is because I live in two worlds. Giving up one world, one identity for the other, takes some work, but when I can do that it makes everything easier. But that's new and it's frightening in a way because it's a space I'm not familiar with. It's good, but it's surprising at times and it's hard to know where firm ground is. Because of my background, that protective part of me is always there. Feeling safe enough is not a common thing for me, but the more I'm able to do that the easier it is to bring my female voice through. But that will always be something I'll have to be conscious of. Not just in singing life, but other parts of life as well.

Int: When you're out performing, how comfortable and confident do you feel in your singer's identity? Do you tend to gravitate toward "boy songs" or "girl songs"?

Regina: In karaoke, I do "boy songs" because if I'm my male self, that's what people expect.

Int: Would you choose differently if you were singing as your female self?

Regina: Oh for sure, and I have. I'll sing different songs because I want to as Regina. I pick different songs, absolutely. As a woman, I don't feel that I want to sing male songs, though a lot of women sing male songs. I'm just not driven in that direction. There have been times I've sung female songs as a male, but people look at me quizzically. Cis women can sing men's songs and people are comfortable with that, but a man singing a woman's song really makes people uncomfortable. If I'm in my male self, I'll tend to sing male songs, but I'll try to push it a little. As Regina, I want to sing Regina songs. I can't say I've never done boy songs, but I wouldn't be driven to do that. So quick answer is: if I'm Regina I try to do songs that Regina always would've wanted to do.

Int: Do you think that being able to spend more time as Regina has changed the way you inhabit yourself? Do you think that's affected your connection to that part of you, especially as a singer?

Regina: There are times I reorient my life to force more space for Regina because it's almost like a competition for the time. In the past, there have been times when I had to really deliberately make room for that. I've become an officer in a trans social group because it forces me to go there every month, forces me to be involved. I took formal dancing lessons once, partly just because I love it, and because it forces me to bring out more of Regina. Voice lessons are similar, so it affects me, but that doesn't stop my life from pulling me toward my male self as well. I'm an upbeat person, but if I weren't it could be depressing. In a way, how can I say this? If I didn't stop myself I would cry about it. If someone said, "What do you need to do to be really happy?" I'd have to split off into two people, which I can't, so I do what I can each way. I'm fortunate in that whatever Regina things I do, my wife is completely open. She's completely fine with it and she never—which is kind of weird—none of it shakes her. None of it. So, I want to do this Regina thing better, I want to have a girl voice.

Int: And singing is obviously a huge part of finding that happiness and balance, in all aspects of your life. What brings you the most freedom and joy in singing?

Regina: That's really difficult to answer because it's emotional. I am happiest when I'm singing. It could be at home, but I'm even happier in front of people. If you do it right, it's your soul coming through with your voice. Not everyone sings that way in my opinion. Some people are very mechanical, but I do think what people take away when they hear me sing is that they're hearing my soul. I think that's what they're connecting to, and I love that. Someone needs to feel it. It's passion. It's not really different for my male or female self except that they inhabit a different part of me, so the feeling is the same but it's felt in a different place. If ever I sang to someone and they didn't emotionally feel it, that would bother me, something wasn't authentic about what I did.

Int: Can you talk a bit about negotiating between these different parts of yourself, in terms of how you approach learning to sing?

Regina: It's very difficult because for the most part, when I struggle with things, I struggle in my other life, and I'm good at struggling but there are things that I do to get through that in my other life. I've struggled with things in my Regina life as well but sadly, often, I pull Etienne, [my male self,] in to get through that because Etienne is very good at that. Growing up where I did, in a really rough place, I had to learn how to protect myself. There are a lot of things I learned in order to thrive in that environment, but those were all as my male self. So as Regina, I have some coping things that I do but if it gets too difficult, I call upon what I'm used to. So going into singing, subconsciously or unconsciously, Etienne shows up for that and I know now that it's not the best way to go about that, but that's the struggle.

Int: Do you notice when it happens?

Regina: No. If I'm paying attention I do, but I think the only thing that will help is time, and my teacher pointing that out in time.

Int: Do you think being able to spend more time singing as Regina and inhabiting that voice will help, too?

Regina: Sure, and being aware. Once you're aware you can address it. I've come to believe that we're not as in charge of ourselves as we think we are. Your brain does a whole lot of things without your consent. And so, I think that when I'm at a loss, the other brain says, "Do this thing, it will keep you safe" but it hasn't asked my consent. For me, I think there's just a whole lot of things to work through, and one of them is being aware and being comfortable. Over the years, I've met people who were closeted trans people and they were just caught in their own fear. They'd come to a group meeting where all these trans people are, and they would sit in the car for a half hour because they're afraid to go in. They would drive around for a while and then just go home because they're so frightened by the possibilities, because it's so new. Someone said to me once that she dressed up as a woman, and when she looked in the mirror she looked so good to herself, so much more like herself, that she didn't do it again for years because it frightened the other part of her, to see that her female identity might be real. Anything that's new is a little frightening, so inhabiting the Regina voice is not devoid of fear. I don't overplay that, but you find yourself thrilled and uncomfortable at the same time. It feels odd and strange and I want to do more, but it's going deeper into the rabbit hole. Certainly, there's much less risk in my life today than there was, but there's still the potential, again, for anyone who's different. If someone finds out that you're not who they think you are, and there's that loss of trust towards you, you risk the loss of affection from the people around you. Whenever you're different, there's always a concern about behaving appropriately for whatever the situation is.

Int: How do you think that affects the way you use your voice?

Regina: I was thinking about this on the way here today, and I think generally speaking in short bursts, my voice is good enough. I go everywhere and no one seems to be shocked or taken aback so I don't worry much about it. I think I'm blessed in that I can come and go. Out of all the years, maybe twice I've been worried about it. Once, I was with a friend at a train convention, and this person is trans, but she was there as a boy. She had a female friend with her and she introduced me to her friend, and her friend said, "Oh I love your hair, who does your hair?" And it's a wig, of course. So I was afraid of outing my friend through this conversation, because now she's introduced me as a girlfriend of hers, and I don't want to—

Int: And you didn't know if the other friend knew that your friend is trans, and if you got clocked it might accidentally out your friend—

Regina: Absolutely. But I think it went fine, but that's when I might be worried about my voice. But I think the lessons have helped me inhabit my female voice better, yes. It's difficult for me, though, and probably always will be unless I drop a bunch of things and just focus on that, but that's hard to do because I'm still in this other chorus as my male self. I think, I guess I'd say this: There are times you take what's given to you. I can be better, but probably not as good as I could've been if I could truly devote my time. Lots of people want to get better with their voice, but they won't do it, they're afraid of it, or they don't want to do the work, but nothing comes without all that. I'll at least go down the path. I think I'm that person. I won't let the fear stop me, or I won't dwell on all these reasons it won't work out. In the group I'm in, I sing tenor, but I stand next to the altos and sometimes I sing their part and they look at me, you know sideways. And I can sing the soprano part, and they look at me as if to say, "Why would you even do that?" but I like it, I enjoy it. I think that's just related to conforming—people love, or want, to conform. I'm not so good at it.

Int: Can you talk a little more about your choral experience? Choirs can be such heavily gendered spaces. Has that ever made you uncomfortable?

Regina: Does it make me uncomfortable? No, it hasn't made me uncomfortable, but I recognize it's a rule. The payoff of challenging that rule is low, and the risk is high. I could sing some other part, but the general feeling is that we have women who do soprano and alto, and men that do bass and tenor, and that's what we do. Let's say I wanted to push the envelope, to perform as Regina, and I wanted to be in the alto section. I could probably do it but there would be some fallout somewhere, and so the question for me is whether it would be worth the fallout. Singing tenor is hard enough! And I think if someone were to argue against me singing alto, they would say, "Sure, you could do the alto part, but could you do it as well as altos we already have?"

Int: What would make that environment more welcoming for you? How do you think that environment is different from something like an all-trans choir?

Regina: When I first heard about Resonate, I thought, "What a wonderful idea, I could perform again as Regina." And I knew that other people could choose to express themselves however they wanted and now have the opportunity to that. I was thrilled about it, and a little frightened, because it would be new. Resonate is taking another step toward normalizing [trans] people, and I think that's what a lot of [cis] people don't like. You are who you are, however you call yourself whether it's female, male, or whatever it is. This is who you are, this is what you want to do and if you can do it, what more is there to talk about? The more people are exposed to [trans identities], the less weird it is to them. Which is, of course, why people want to go back the old way, because it's becoming too normalized.

Int: What do you think are some of the ways you've been limited or influenced by someone else's expectations about gender, about what's "normal"?

Regina: You know stereotypically, men mask their emotion in their voice, they mask them because they don't want you to know how they really feel. Women stereotypically give it to you, and even say, "This is how I feel, I'm going to cry." Men are generally not going to do that. Sometimes I'll do that and people, again, look at me funny. Because I watch movies, I'll just cry. My daughter won't cry, but *I'll* cry. Something happens and she'll look over at me and say, "Are you crying?" and I'll say *(in a low, gruff voice)* "uhh, I'm not crying" but I'll cry. That's not normally something you announce to people. There have been times where I've been in public and I'll start to cry, and so I'll try not to, because people look at me kind of funny then.

Int: Does that ever show up in your singing, those differences in emotional candor or emotional availability?

Regina: When I sing, I have to control it, because if you go too far down that path people start to look at you. I think a cis woman has more room to maneuver emotionally than a cis male. Like, there are times [as my male self] I'll say to women, "Oh I really love your hair," or I'll say, "That's a really nice blouse you have on" because that's what I'm thinking, but men don't normally do that unless they're leading somewhere else. If I'm singing, in some way singing is the root of Regina. That isn't to say that all that Etienne stuff isn't in there, but as Regina, you could argue the singing is more authentic except that there's all the Etienne mechanics in there. But it's just emotions and it's hard to sort it out. I would argue that even— when I started singing, I sang in a falsetto with a very feminine style. I was drawn to that and I didn't start singing differently until I started joining these choruses, and I miss that voice, so lately I've been working more on that head voice.

Int: Was there ever someone who questioned that style? Who questioned why you were using your high voice like that?

Regina: Someone said that to me just recently. I was singing the women's part in this group and the person who sits next to me was asking me why I did that and I said, "Well I used to always sing that way," and she said, "Why did you sing that way?" Like why would I do that, you know? And I just said, "Well that was my voice," and I told her I didn't start singing this way until recently, pretty much when I joined the group.

Int: Why did you change your voice?

Regina: Well, because that's what's called for in the chorus.

Int: Do you think if you hadn't been put in the tenor part and expected to sing that way that you'd still be singing high?

Regina: Oh yeah, that's my preferred singing. I enjoy the tenor singing because it stretches me and gives me another thing on the résumé, but if given the choice, I'd sing the other way, just because that's my preference. Back in the dark ages, the '70s and such, there were a lot of falsetto singers. But then came a time when the rap started up and you had to be more boisterous and manly, so people had the expectation that you'd sing more like that. So, in order to exist or fit in I thought I needed to be more versatile. I don't regret it, but when I started singing more that way I kind of lost my old voice. Voice lessons have helped me with that, and the mechanics help me, but Etienne and Regina are mixed up in me. I think at the root, I want to express the emotion. I want to sing the emotional songs, the love songs, that kind of thing. I think the root of that is Regina, but even in doing more challenging songs, I think I was bringing more of Regina into that.

Int: Anything else you'd like to say about your voice?

Regina: I think it's more of a journey for me than for other people voice-wise, but I would say the biggest benefit of lessons has been, in general, that the mechanics help me no matter how I'm singing. The thing we've explored a bit, bringing out the Regina voice, there hasn't been much progress because it's a harder road, a bumpier road. I sing so much to begin with, that challenges my voice. Now, having to do this other thing that challenges it even more, sometimes it's worrisome, but it's worth it because I love to sing.

Int: Thank you, Regina.

Regina: My pleasure!

MJ

MJ is an amateur singer who performs in a choral group, at several local karaoke bars, and with her company rock band. She is also a programmer and engineer, and holds a master's degree in linguistics. She is especially adept at soaking up concepts around voice anatomy and function and integrating them with her background to refine the use of her voice both in speaking and singing. MJ also supports several online groups as they maneuver their own voice journeys and is always seeking more knowledge to support her communities.

MJ is simultaneously bubbly and deeply thoughtful, vivacious, and nurturing. Her performance life has grown during her time in lessons from shyly considering a few sung notes in a previously limited range to fronting bands for several performances and writing her own music, complete with vocal improvisations and lush harmonies. MJ's journey is inspiring and she has a great deal to offer with her fun and casual analysis of gender theory as it relates to voice. In this interview, she discusses how some of her education in philosophy and linguistics affects the way she feels about her voice and about how the world at large views gender and voice.

Int: indicates the interviewers

MJ: indicates the student's response

Int: We're here with MJ, and it's a crisp fall day.

MJ: That's right, that's right, I have some tea. Feeling pretty chill.

Int: Feeling pretty good.

MJ: Oh yeah.

(laughter)

Int: So, talk a little bit about your singing life.

MJ: Oh, OK, yeah, love that question. I've been working hard at my singing, mostly in the form of being a member of Resonate, which is a trans choir in Chicago, been doing that for about a year and a half, almost going on 2 years. That was the first time I've actually sung outside of mumbling stuff at church or whatever.

Int: And you've been taking lessons for about as long, too. Why did you decide to start singing lessons and join the choir?

MJ: I was walking down the street, because I live near the studio, and I just saw the sign and it had that sort of . . . presage . . . feeling? Anyway, what preceded the decision to take lessons was wanting to do more singing. I was the friend who kept wanting to go to the karaoke bar, and I was at the early stages of transition, and I really like singing. Even so, I wasn't super comfortable and I thought I should learn how to sing. I mean, blending or passing is a fraught concept, but I didn't want to be read as a boy in my day-to-day life, and especially in my voice life and in my singing life. I thought, "If I'm going to I learn to talk in a way that's more congruent, I'm going learn to sing in a way that's more congruent." I also just want to learn how to sing, because I want to do this well. And everything came together.

Int: And then Resonate started. What was that like for you?

MJ: My first impression coming into Resonate rehearsals or auditions or whatever was like, "Holy crap, there are other people who want to sing! There are people like me who want learn how to use their voices!" I had a lot of enthusiasm, but not a lot of formal background in singing. I'm working really hard at that, but also at the same time, the kinds of songs I want to sing are not usually songs which are sung in my register. It's been a process of unlearning gendered expectations, it's been a process of learning how to use my voice, and it's been a process of learning what it is about music or about singing that I really enjoy. When I first started, I had this naive idea that I would just learn how to sing, and I'd be done.

Int: Just like that.

MJ: Just like that, well, great, I'll just learn to sing, and I'll be great. But of course, with anything complex and interesting, there are levels within levels and nuance within nuance. But singing opens up more opportunities to engage with people and engage with myself. I kind of shut down creatively around high school, so I'm gradually finding new ways of creating and it's a slow process, but it's been really useful. Now my voice life is rich, and it's varied and busy, and I feel like I don't have enough time in the day to fit in all the voice things I want to do.

Int: Can you say a little more about shutting down creatively in high school?

MJ: There isn't a whole lot to this story, it's just that I used to draw and write a lot when I was in middle school, and then in high school, I was afraid of the things that I was pulled towards, and I didn't want to seem . . . it was like . . . How do I . . . I haven't thought about it super deeply in a really long time, but basically I was afraid of the things that I was drawn towards producing. The things that motivated my heart or my visual art started fading a little bit as I got into high school. I just felt aimless, like I was flailing around, and I think part of it was definitely me running away from things that were signs that I was trans. I lost my view, so to speak, because the things that I did want to write about or create weren't cool comic book things. I went to an all boys' high school, and I felt like I was languishing and was pulled away from artistic outlets. With art, music, writing, and so forth, I lost my inspiration for creation. I wanted to write about being a girl, and I formed artistic role models through TV characters or pop culture figures, but they weren't supposed to be my artistic role models because I was supposed to be a boy. If I had pursued it more, I might have found a way to keep my artistic voice during that time, but I didn't understand myself, and I didn't want to. So singing again now, this is just making me understand myself.

Int: And it sounds like you have been able to rekindle some of that artistic expression?

MJ: Yeah, I am able to rekindle a little bit of that. And I'm still trying to discover the tools that I have for creating without feeling too helpless in trying to relearn how to create. I'm a little scared of it, but I see possibilities unfurling, which is good.

Int: How do you think voice lessons and singing in Resonate have impacted that?

MJ: Well, certainly it has reduced the level of guilt and fear of myself and what I can do and what I can produce. It has given me space to explore things in a technical way that is also pleasing to me. And those seem like small things, but they're not. There's significance in something as straightforward as singing a song together, with all the attention to detail, and the communal creative process that comes from people being in sync with each other. It's liberating because I'm no longer competing with people to be the most technically proficient or the best in some way. It's awesome to be around people who are like me, who aren't as sure of themselves, and are as new as me. In that space, there's only room for support, and no room for dismissal or comparing or competition.

Int: When you were in high school, did you find yourself measuring your art against other people?

MJ: Oh, for sure. It would be like, "Oh, you can draw? Can you draw *this*?" And comparing or competing becomes the meaning of what we're doing. But in Resonate, it's a chance to rethink that, to see that the creating comes from somewhere else and has a different meaning. It's not, "Oh you can sing? Can you sing *this*?" There's just never that element.

Int: You mentioned being able to explore technically as well as artistically. How do you think your application of techniques and skills has fed your own sense of creating beauty and music?

MJ: I think of someone like Ella Fitzgerald, a really amazing singer with an equally amazing songbook. The level of access that I had to that starting out was mostly focused on the lyrics, and some tone quality, and rhythm. I could make passing observations about how she hit the notes or how interesting the song was because those were the features that were most accessible. Learning more about singing gives me appreciation and understanding about more complex attributes, like the choices she might have made as an artist. I'm able to perceive the creative aspects of singing, and strive for that complexity in my own music. I guess it's like having dawning awareness of that stuff. It makes me a more nuanced critic and I'm more aware of where my taste is going for my own art. It's like a redefinition and focusing of my taste, and I can look at music that I always loved and appreciate it in a new way. And I can start to feel it if I want to mimic it, and I have tools to help me try it out.

Int: You're also passionate about the science of singing, since you have a background in linguistics. How has your unique skillset and way of perceiving and practicing technique affected your learning process?

MJ: Well, it's always a work in progress. It's one thing to know the acoustic and articulatory properties of a vowel but it's different to think about how to change the vowel to make a different color or sound. And what I find interesting is there is this kind of, not prescriptive, but there's utility to that knowledge now when it comes to singing, which is fun to connect to.

Int: How has your knowledge of linguistics and acoustics influenced your singing voice in a gendered way? How do you use those tools to find your "authentic" singing voice?

MJ: I wish I knew. I mean, is there a way? I wish there was a system of levels, like once you figure out one thing you move on to the next. But it's a constant process, a push-and-pull of applying and acquiring knowledge. But I think it does help me practically in some ways, knowing how similar voices can be, and how much overlap there is between perceived gender in different voices. Philosophy has also been a really great help to me. I studied philosophy as an undergrad in college. One of the things that stuck with me is how easy it is to impose pretheoretical assumptions and biases on the world; to assume that because there is a difference in my mind, and I observe that difference out in the world, that it means that what I see in my mind is validated and reinforced by the state of the world. And I think that same thing applies to voice. We observe differences between male and female voices, and we have this distinction in our minds, so because they're very distinct categories in our minds, and we see them in the world, it must mean it's true—there must be fundamental difference in the world. This doesn't take into account any of the vast overlap, and it doesn't take into account the concept of a spectrum or a continuum. And in linguistics, it's easy to impose categorical structure on continuous phenomena. I remember learning about speech perception and we did an exercise in creating blends of [s] and [ʃ], and asked listeners to make a judgment about which sound something is more similar to. The stimuli were continuous, but those judgments, it's like at some point, at the midpoint, they just flipped. That property of our brains to impose categories is interesting, and we can't help it. So, for my voice, I'm aware that I have to get to a certain point across the midline in order for people's judgments to flip from male to female when they hear me.

Int: What a great point! If male and female are the only options that exist in our mind, and then those mutually exclusive categories are reinforced by observations about the world, it leaves us blind to all the in-between and all the gray area. And the reality is most voices fall into that gray space, somewhere.

MJ: Absolutely. If we live in a continuous world, to what degree do I even need to impose this categorical ordering? Maybe it's awesome living in the gray space. . . . But it's easier to get by when people can fit you into the binary because people tend to have a really hard time with incongruence. But, knowing that, I have room to decide if I'm changing my voice for my own sanity's sake, or to just make it easier to get by day to day. Everything is continuous, and it's also categorical, and those categories are not wholly true. So maybe I can perform within these categories for a purpose, but I don't have to buy into them. All of that helps me feel more at home with myself and more at ease about my voice and about my physiology.

Int: You have a lot of knowledge about your own vocal anatomy and physiology, too. How does knowing that impact the way you feel about your voice?

MJ: My vocal anatomy is unique, and it falls in some distribution somewhere. The size of my larynx, the prominence of my thyroid notch, the thickness of my vocal cords, are all unique and apparently somewhere in the middle. And that makes me feel like maybe I don't have to work so hard to get people to flip that judgment about my voice. I have been experimenting with trying to sing with my larynx lower than I have allowed myself to do in the past, and that's been interesting and kind of fun. I can try and incorporate that information, and let myself relax a little and not feel like it's as risky.

Int: You were talking about things that you do with your voice that are for you, and things you do that are for other people. Can you talk a little bit about some of the choices

you make as a singer that are just for you, and whether those choices feel risky because of how they will be heard?

MJ: Yes, the audience that I'm totally comfortable with is myself. The only audience that I trust completely and utterly to not react terribly. . . .

Int: And when you say, "react terribly," what does that mean?

MJ: Worst-case scenario would be physical violence. What I'm afraid of is involuntarily being gendered the wrong way, which has social ramifications. If someone hears me and starts thinking, "Oh, you're a dude, that means you don't actually belong with us, and we're not hanging out with you, and everything you ever said is going to be retroactively re-judged and reassessed in light of the way we see you now because you lied to us." Like, I'm afraid of being accused explicitly, or treated implicitly, as though I've somehow been deceptive or inauthentic. Which is, of course, the opposite of what I want to be. I feel this very strong need to protect my history, because I'm never sure how it's going to be used, and that also extends to the people who know me the most. It feels like gender is so central to how we assess and categorize and decide who our friends are and who the strangers are. I'm constantly afraid that all of a sudden, I could go from being in the friend category to the stranger category. And the closer the person is to me, the greater the risk of being retroactively and irrevocably reassigned to stranger as opposed to friend, companion, somebody you thought you understood. So that's really for me the risk.

Int: That's a pretty big risk. How do you make choices, then, that balance both of those things?

MJ: Yeah, there are certain parts of my range that I think sound more female, and will get gendered more correctly than other parts of my range. And the low part of my range is something that I'm trying to fit in. But I only practice that on my own a little bit. I feel very self-conscious about performing there. Even parts of my high range make me self-conscious. When I pick songs that I'll end up performing, I tend to pick things that camp out squarely in the middle. I'm still figuring out how to approach different parts of my range. There are definitely male artists that sing in ranges that overlap with female singers, but often they do it in a way that's stereotypically masculine. I'm learning now about how I would approach those songs and what's interesting is that I feel like in the past, I didn't worry about being too loud, but now it's like even if I try to be loud in that range, I don't quite know how. I get caught in this conundrum where I know the song well and it works well with my range, but it's sung by a boy, and I have to ask myself, "How would I sing that? How are people expecting me to sing that?" I feel like I should sing the artists. But if I sing at karaoke or something, are people wondering why I'm singing a boy song? Or why I'm not singing the girl songs? I feel that sometimes, like I'll sing like an Elton John song or something, and people react to that like it's strange.

Int: What is that like, when you get that reaction?

MJ: I mean, it's kind of flipped, it used to be that people were weirded out if I sang a girl song, and now they're weirded out if I sing a boy song. It's not a bad thing, I'm still trying to work out that reaction.

Int: Do you think that's a form of gender policing?

MJ: I wonder if it is, yeah. Of course, it could all be in my head, but I think it's a legitimate thing. Even if I sing a girl song terribly, that seems to be better than if I sing a boy song pretty well.

Int: Have you experienced any other policing about your gender?

MJ: There are some people who really want to sing high, but there's also some people saying, "I'm a girl, but I'm going to sing low." I would say in the do-it-yourself trans voice community, like on Reddit and other online groups, there is this desire to go super high, and there is a little competition around "Well I can hit a G," "Well I can hit a high C."

Int: Do you think that's mostly intra-community, or do you think that comes from somewhere else?

MJ: I don't know, I mean, we're all prisoners of gender. We've all absorbed the same messages about what femininity is and is not. We all know that all girls are supposed to sing high and boys are supposed to sing low. And if you're a boy who sings high, that's bad, and if you're a girl who sings low, that's not great either unless you're willing to sing tenor, then that's good, because most boys don't want to sing tenor parts. But for us, I think there's a sense that we're proving ourselves, and we have to prove ourselves all the time. We're all pretty familiar with gendered expectations, but different people enforce them in different ways and take that to different extremes. I do think that we tend to go out of our way to show, "I can be really feminine! And really a girl, for real! Believe me!" That comes from the real world that we're trying to traverse, all the time. It's probably just amplified a little bit. For me, I just want to be a girl, but how do you be the girl that is me, when I have so many examples of girls who are *not* me? And I don't know what to do. And I don't know what my voice is. And sometimes I just want someone to tell me what to do! We all have to be professional gender theorists, but I just want to live my life.

Int: How do you think we could equip teachers to be the gender theory experts so that their students don't have to be?

MJ: I think there is defensive gender theory and exploratory, playful gender theory. Defensive gender theory involves learning how to adequately defend my choices against the world, to shield my identity from onslaught and carry that shield at all times. Exploratory gender theory is more about being a fellow traveler, about being curious about your own gender while I'm exploring and unveiling mine. It's useful for teachers to be able to articulate some of the key concepts in a way that's protective and gives people a safe place to explore. When teachers rely on students to be the gender experts, it puts students on the defensive and it makes them try to explain different aspects of gender for the sake of protecting their own identities. And then it's hard to get them to explore and experiment artistically if they feel constantly at risk or under scrutiny about their identity. I want [teachers] to know enough to protect and affirm their students, and keep the students from having to defend themselves. The voice lesson should be a place where they don't have to defend anything. There are moments where the student may not know that they're being too critical of themselves, but they're also saying that because they expect that's how the world is going to see them.

Int: Have there been times in your voice education when your teachers have failed you, or put you on the defensive about your identity?

MJ: No, I mean, I'm very lucky with my voice education, specifically around trans voice. I have a nurturing and very safe environment there. But it's also just the world at large.

Int: You have such a strong connection with your community; what are some instances where you have seen other voice professionals who might have failed your community?

MJ: I think that there are assumptions people make about range or preferred vocal style, and assumptions about whether a song is "right." I see snap judgments about where a person should sing, as opposed to where they want to sing. Maybe there's a misconception that part of what a voice teacher is supposed to do is size you up and say, "Well you should sing here because . . . " whatever xyz reason. I would like to see teachers take a step back and reevaluate how those judgments are formulated and whether they need to be static. We're so willing to assign people in static categories, and it happens unconsciously and without malice, but it's so ingrained. It will take work on both the teacher and students' parts.

Int: How have your voice educators supported you and your community in the ways you needed it?

MJ: I think one really useful thing is checking in pretty frequently about voice goals. That process of reassessment is super helpful, and permitting progress in a particular direction, even if a goal seems far-fetched, is great. Allowing a person to make their own decisions about what they really want to achieve is helpful. And I guess the other thing is trying to open up, when a goal might be very hard maybe there's a compromise somewhere. Voice range is so important to a lot of people, but if someone has a goal about their range that isn't achievable yet or something, getting to the root of that goal is helpful. Maybe there's another way to work towards it through developing resonance or articulation, or releasing some tension, to pave the way to come back to that big goal later. But really, just being with the student and validating and supporting their goals, while being open to compromise and alternatives, is super important.

Int: What do you want to say to trans and nonbinary students who are interested in learning about themselves?

MJ: I would say trust yourself. I would say that your voice has depths and possibilities that are probably way beyond where you first imagine them, even if you have an extensive vocal background. We're still learning, and you can really give back, if you choose. Everything you learn can be used to help others, and we're all taking first steps along this path, which is pretty exciting and amazing. And nobody knows anything! Anybody who tells you that you can't do something is probably wrong.

Int: Probably definitely wrong.

MJ: Probably definitely wrong, right? And if you figure something out, awesome!

Int: Anything else you want to say?

MJ: Chill out the larynx.

Int: *(laughing)* **Chill out with the larynx-raising!**

MJ: *(laughing)* I don't know, thank you for giving me a chance to rant and ramble.

Int: We're honored to share your story.

APPENDIX

1

Sample Student Intake Form

NEW STUDENT INFORMATION SHEET

Student Preferred Name: _____

Pronouns: _____

Parent/guardian if under 18: _____

Address: _____ Apt: _____

City: _____ State: _____ Zip: _____

Phone: _____ Email: _____

Voice History Information

Are you currently participating in hormone therapy treatment? _____

If yes, please describe type(s), dosage, frequency, and length of treatment:

_____

Have you had any operations that would affect your voice? (laryngoplasty, rhinoplasty, facial feminization surgery, voice feminization surgery)?

_____

Have you ever taken voice lessons or received voice training?   YES   NO

If yes, please describe:

_____

_____

Have you ever had problems with your voice? i.e., chronic hoarseness, sore throat, long periods of laryngitis, hemorrhage, nodules, cysts, polyps, or other lesions.

YES   NO

If yes, please describe:

_____

_____

Do you smoke?   YES   NO

What are your goals for voice training?

_____

_____

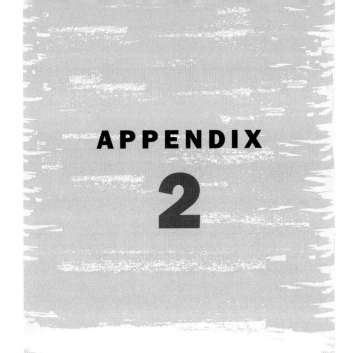

APPENDIX

2

Transgender Inclusive and Affirming Policies

SAMPLE POLICY EXCERPTS

Students at private studios, universities, and other institutions need support systems to feel safe and thrive in their learning environments. Included in this appendix is sample language to guide administrative teams in the creation of updated school policies to include trans and nonbinary students. Trans-affirming policies should include sections about terminology, discrimination, use of preferred name and pronouns, supporting students during transition, classroom and choral behavior expectations, dress code, facility access, parental/guardian involvement, and professional development/training.

Terminology

Refer to Chapter 1 for a detailed list of terminology relevant to supporting trans and nonbinary students. Basic terminology for institutional policies should include terms that explain some of the different iterations of gender identity and gender expression.

Discrimination

It is the policy of (Institution Name) to prohibit discrimination or bullying based on sex, sexual orientation, gender identity, or gender expression. Any act of discrimination, whether committed by faculty, staff, or a fellow student, will receive immediate attention, investigation, and action, appropriate to the scenario. Enforcement will focus on education and support rather than exclusionary discipline.

Preferred Name and Pronouns

Students have the right to be addressed by the name and pronouns that align with their gender identity. (Institution Name) allows students to use their preferred name and gender pronouns, regardless of whether legal procedures to change their name and pronouns have arisen. Teachers will inquire privately with the student about preferred name and pronouns for use in classroom settings and in communication with parents/guardians. At a time of the student's choosing, name and pronouns can be updated within administrative systems, including school identification, email addresses, class rosters, transcripts, records, etc. All personnel at (Institution Name) will make every effort to use the student's new name and pronouns. Parental/guardian approval is not required for a student to change their name and pronouns at (Institution Name).

Supporting Students During Transition

(Institution Name) accepts the gender identity of a student without resistance or question. There will be no thresholds to this acceptance; the gender identity of a student is valid regardless of social, medical, or legal transition status. Each student's transition is unique and (Institution Name) will support the student in the ways that allow equal access to educational programs and activities, always with the student's safety and success at the fore.

Classroom and Choral Behavior

Fellow students are expected to uphold nondiscriminatory behaviors in choral and classroom settings. Once a choir member has stated their preferred name and pronouns, or if a member chooses to change them, all other members will use the student's new name and pronouns. If one student accidentally uses the wrong name or pronouns for another student, an apology and hasty correction is expected from the student who made the mistake. Although mistakes may happen from time to time, misgendering or misidentifying a fellow student is not tolerated. It is expected that choir and classroom members will advocate for each other and provide a mutually inclusive and supportive environment.

Dress Code

Students have the right to use dress code regulations, costumes, outfits, or other clothing (such as choir robes) that align with their gender identity and expression, and may choose to adopt a gender-neutral appearance when possible. Transgender and gender nonconforming students will not suffer a stricter expectation than cisgender students about dress codes because of their gender identity.

Facility Access

Students may access the restroom, locker room, dressing room, or changing facility in which they feel most comfortable. Under no circumstances will students be forced to use facilities that are incongruent with their gender identity, nor shall any student be asked to use a separate facility because they are transgender or gender nonconforming. If a student is uncomfortable in gender-segregated facilities, a separate, nonstigmatizing option will be available.

Parental/Guardian Involvement

Teachers and staff at (Institution Name) will center the student's needs when considering parental/guardian involvement. Following the student's lead as to when teachers and staff should speak openly about the student's transition at school with parents/guardians, (Institution Name) will offer support to parents by sharing resources and providing a positive example of use of the student's preferred name and pronouns.

GLSEN Model Policy:

"Staff should take guidance from and work collaboratively with the student to ensure that the student remains safe, both at school and at home. This may include, for example: determining what information to share with the student's parents or guardians; identifying resources that could assist the parents or guardians to better understand how to support their child; and, how to communicate with the student's siblings as well as staff and other students." (GLSEN, 2016)

Professional Development/Training

(Institution Name) provides training for teachers and staff to ensure adherence to applicable laws and to this policy. To the extent that resources are available, (Institution Name) will provide continuing education and training for teachers and staff in the realms of terms, concepts, and current understanding of gender identity; communication strategies for students and parents/guardians; curriculum development and classroom management; suicide prevention; responsibilities of teachers, staff, and management.

REFERENCES

California State. (1998). Sex Equity in Education Act. *California Education Code Section §221.5*. (C. 9. 4, Ed.).

DC Public Schools. (2016). *Transgender and gender nonconforming policy guidance*. Washington, DC: DC Public Schools.

GLSEN. (2016). *Model district policy on transgender and gender nonconforming students*. New York, NY: GLSEN, National Center for Transgender Equality.

Vannasdall, D. (2015). *Transgender students—Ensuring equity and nondiscrimination*. Arcadia Unified School District, Superintendent. Arcadia, CA: Arcadia Unified School District.

APPENDIX

3

Voice Exercises

The following exercises may give teachers additional examples of training techniques to guide students through challenges specifically faced by transgender and nonbinary singers.

RESPIRATION (CHAPTER 5)

Trans/nonbinary singers face two potentially significant challenges in developing breath efficiency. Body-shaping garments such as chest binders or waist trainers/corsets may prevent trans singers from taking a full breath. Encourage singers to develop awareness and flexibility in the parts of the body that are not constricted by such garments. Gender dysphoria may cause singers to disconnect from their bodies or find themselves in a state of anxiety or hypervigilance. As students develop awareness of the functions of respiration and body alignment, prefacing new exercises with the phrase "what would it be like to . . . " helps to build trust and ensure agency for the student.

Exercises to develop flexibility and buoyancy in the diaphragm, abdominals, and intercostal muscles benefit the student in singing through the challenges of body-shaping garments. Exercises 5a and 5b should be performed at a moderate or slow tempo, ensuring the student inhales and exhales evenly for the same lengths of time.

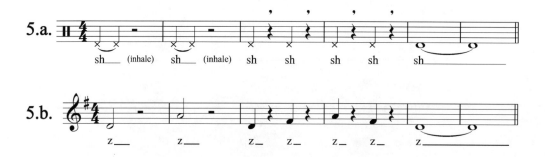

PITCH AND REGISTRATION (CHAPTER 7)

Some singers desire to align their pitch range with their gender identity, but some are comfortable in their current, pretransition voice range. Along with range development, trans masculine singers who choose testosterone hormone therapy may need extra guidance and support in maneuvering register breaks.

Exercises 7a to 7d are intended to develop smooth movement through the passaggi and may be used at varying points along a singer's vocal range. Exercise 7e helps singers develop awareness and control of chest voice and head voice as well as flexibility in navigating register breaks; this exercise can also be used as varying points along the range. Exercise 7f can help singers develop flute register and high head voice. Exercises 7g and 7h help develop strength and flexibility in registers and can be used to develop chest voice.

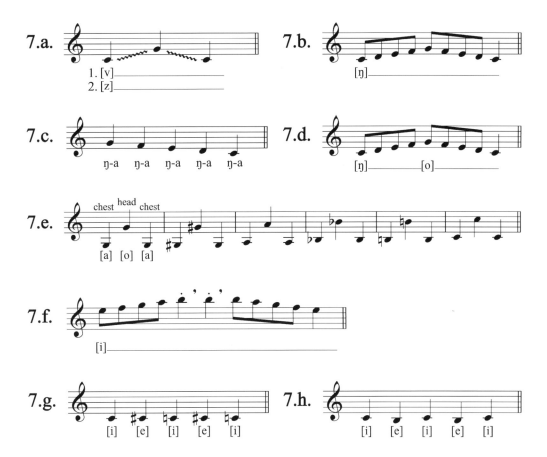

RESONANCE AND ARTICULATION (CHAPTER 8)

Masculinization and feminization of resonance and articulation play an important role in aligning a singer's voice with their gender or influencing an audience to perceive gender in a voice. Exercises in this realm encourage trans masculine singers to create a darker sound with articulation that resides slightly farther back in the mouth or on the tongue, and trans feminine singers to create a brighter sound with very light articulation at the front of the mouth and tip of the tongue. Exercise 8a helps singers perceive and adjust vowel shapes toward a darker, deeper resonance and is helpful for trans masculine singers. Exercise 8b works in the opposite direction to develop brighter resonance for trans feminine singers.

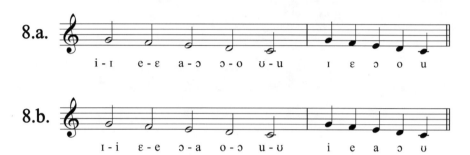

The following tongue twisters can also be used to practice articulation patterns. Students can experiment with articulation that occurs at the back of the mouth, in the middle, and at the very front to discover the patterns and habits that feel the most natural and authentic.

1. Annie is an independent astronomer.
2. Pumpkin pie is not an appropriate pest repellant.
3. Send Sammy sixteen extracts straight away.
4. Fifteen fresh fuchsia flowers fit perfectly.
5. Linda lays lovely lavender.
6. Kendall collects colorful keychains.
7. Shelves of shimmering shapes were touched by torchlight.

PRACTICE ROUTINES

Practice routines for trans singers may vary from other students due to the athletic nature of voice training and to challenges that may arise from vocal dysphoria. Support the students in discovering the best balance of techniques and optimal practice times so that they feel safe exploring and developing new voice habits. Practice routines and lesson plans should include a combination of the following elements:

- Relaxation—rhythmic breathing, movement exercises
- Slow, careful body awareness—body mapping exercises, use of a mirror only if it feels comfortable
- Breath—release breath around body-shaping garments carefully without inducing tension
- Pitch range experimentation—follow the student's lead about comfort level in different areas of the vocal range. Practice steady pitch range extension exercises that engage, but do not rush, the singer.
- Registration—flexibility between registers, strength and stamina in desired registers
- Resonance—exploration and comfort with the sound of one's own voice, exercises for masculinization or feminization (or both) of resonance
- Articulation—techniques for clear diction that guide the singer toward the desired sound
- Musicality—apply technical tools to musical phrases and songs. Develop awareness of different elements of vocal technique that align with the desired result.

INDEX

Note: Page numbers in **bold** reference non-text material.